RAW MAGIC

Kate Magic

Process Media
1240 W Sims Way, #124
Port Townsend, WA 98368
processmediainc.com

Design by Gregg Einhorn
Photos on the following pages by Kate Magic: 76, 85, 86, 89, 91, 95, 107, 109, 110, 113, 118, 121, 122, 125, 128, 131, 137, 143, 145, 148, 150, 155, 156, 163, 165, 175, 181, 183, 184, 195, 197, 200, 207, 208, 213, 215, 221, 223, 224, 226, 231, 234, 239, 244, 251.

ISBN 978-1-934170-37-3

Printed in The United States of America

1 2 3 4 5 6 7 8 9 10

RAW MAGIC
Superfoods for Superpeople

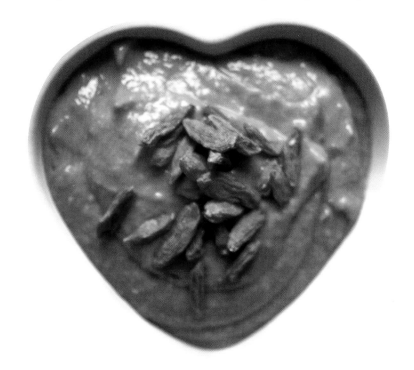

Kate Magic

PROCESS

Contents

Acknowledgements

These are a few of the people I am blessed to know and be inspired by: Reuben, Ethan, Zachary, Chris, Dani, Hudro, Red & Dan, Amy, Solla, Ani, Tonya, Ysanne, Annie, Urduja, Boris, Anna, Julia, Caroline, Nicolas, Erica, Soren, George, Jónsi & Alex, Alfred, Benji, Gilles, Charlie, Amelia, BA, Jo. If you think you should have been on this list and I omitted you, you're probably right; I did so for the sake of brevity, not because I don't love you.

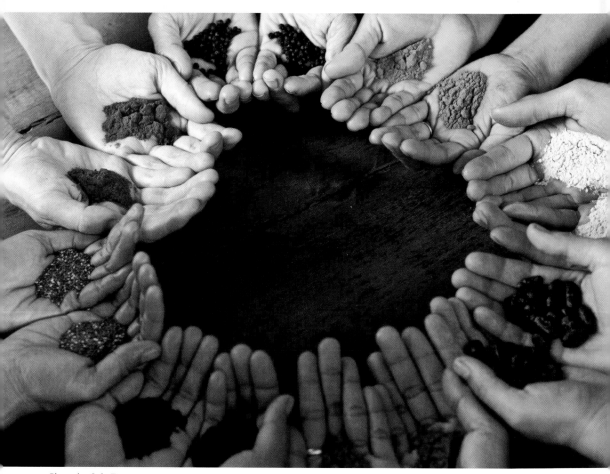

Photo by Suki Zoe

What is Raw Magic?

There are some foods that have the power to change your life.

There are certain foods that when you eat them, your body is in heaven, your cells start singing, your mind becomes ecstatic. "Yes," they cry in unison, "Yes, these are the foods that I have been waiting for. These are the foods that I have been craving, that my body has been missing my whole life." Sometimes, it is a particular nutrient you have been lacking. But more often with these foods it is their synergistic properties. They have a magical energy that comes not only from the synergy of their nutritional composition but from the way they are grown, the lands they are from, their history. Many of them are sacred plants in their countries of origin.

There are many amazing foods I have omitted from this book, foods that are more commonly recognized as superfoods: vegetables like broccoli, kale and cucumbers, fruits like cranberries, blueberries and grapefruit, sprouts like lentils, sunflower or alfalfa. I was tempted to include avocados and olives, buckwheat and oats, all foods I eat on a daily basis.

But these are foods that most of us are familiar with, and if you are not then there are plenty of books out there that do cover them. This book is about the new breed of superfoods that are unique to the West in the 21st century. Never before have we had access to such a wide variety of plant foods. Some of them we are accustomed to in different forms, like cacao; others have been around for a few decades now, like spirulina; some are widely known in their country of origin, but novel to Europe and the U.S., like goji berries; and some others are utterly brand new to us, like purple corn extract. When I was a child, avocados and kiwis were considered exotic; now they are standard fare in every shopping basket. I believe that such is the potency and vitality of the foods in this book that as people catch on to them, they are going to revolutionize the way we eat, shop and live.

These foods are transformative. By eating such high-potency foods they change the very nature of our reality. They affect our consciousness and raise our energetic level to a degree that has profound implications in all areas of our lives. It is not possible to eat these foods on a daily basis and not feel altered. We live in a culture that is intrinsically false; fueled on junk food, media lies, false gods and political whores, we have forgotten how to be our true selves. These foods help us realign, connect with who we really are, and tune into our higher selves. The more we eat this way, the more we live in our power. This can be a hard adjustment to make in a world where the individual is fundamentally disempowered. Revealing our inner core is usually painful; as we let the masks of self-deception slip away, we have to let go of people and life situations which have been holding us back and preventing us being fully who we are. It is a scary thing to do, to step into our truth and reclaim our birthright when we have been taught our whole lives to avoid truth at all costs, to keep up the façades and not rock the boat. But the more of us who make these choices, the easier it becomes. And what's more, the more we attract into our lives people who have made the same choices and appreciate us for who we honestly are.

Rocking the boat is what we are here to do! Isn't it exciting and exhilarating when you stand up for what you truly believe in? Our time has come, and the old ways are not working anymore. Paradigms are crumbling and new ones are rising in their place. As we understand eternal truths, we see the world for what it is, and understand how desperately things need to change. We align with our higher purpose, the divine intelligence, and see what our life's path is. What mission have we been given? What is our role here at this time? It is to wake the world up, to guide humanity through the massive shifts and changes that are taking place. And of course, that starts with ourselves. We must awaken ourselves. We must keep the balance between being masters of our own reality, taking full responsibility for our lives as a manifestation of our own inner state of being; and being of service, helping to awaken the sleeping masses, and doing everything we can to help people through these times. And you know what the best part is? It's fun. Believe it or not, the universe actually wants us to be happy, it doesn't want us to suffer. And the more we work with the universe, the happier we become, the less we suffer.

We are used to a duality in our minds over food. When I grew up, I had issues around my weight. I was trapped in a no-win situation. I could either eat and feel fat and sluggish, or I could not eat and feel clear and light, but spaced out and weak. As most teenagers do, I was worried about how I looked. I fluctuated between liking the look of my body and feeling happy about myself by not eating, or satisfying my instinctive biological need for food, but not really liking myself. I turned to drugs to help me see my way out of this duality, to escape into an artificially induced state of oneness and bliss. The chemicals I put into my body for years didn't do me any favors physically. But they did open me up to a higher state of being, an understanding that I could experience life the way I wanted to. I understood that my life's path involved trying to find ways to recreate those highs naturally, to adopt lifestyle choices that could assist me in living in my highest truth. I turned to raw foods and yoga, and have been working with those disciplines for over two decades now. I can honestly say the process has been revelatory. It has been an arduous and at times painful journey, but the results just keep coming, and they keep getting better and better. Every time I am opened up to a whole new level of being in myself it blows me away.

This journey is like peeling back layers of an onion. You peel back one layer, you make improvements in your diet by adding certain foods and cutting out others, make changes in your lifestyle to move closer to having the life you really want. For a while you feel amazing, on top of the world. But then you uncover a whole other layer of issues, another set of physical, emotional and mental blocks to work through that had been lying hidden deep within you, but are now out and exposed because you have peeled off the rubbish that had been covering them. This process never stops, it is the path we follow as humans, and the more we are in it, the more we learn to love it, to accept it all, not to resist but to enjoy it all, the ups and the downs; the pain and the pleasure are equal gifts, two sides of the same coin.

So how can foods have such a powerful transformative effect? Thanks to films like *What the Bleep?* and *The Secret*, and books like *The Hidden Messages in Water*, people are beginning to fully grasp the concept Buddha taught us, "With our thoughts we make the world." Everything is energy, and everything is connected. Every thought we have, every action we take, affects the quantum field. The universe is a living breathing intelligent mass and we are inextricably a part of it. If we focus on something long and hard, we affect the quantum field. If we tell the universe over and over, "I haven't got a boyfriend, I haven't got a boyfriend," what's the result? No boyfriend. If we replace that with, "I am attracting a beautiful loving nurturing relationship into my life," result? Result. The skill is in maintaining that focus and intent when the spanner gets thrown into the works, when we have to deal with the stuff that we manifested for ourselves without realising pops its handsome head up. Every single food in this book gives us a boost to such a degree that we feel noticeably better about ourselves. When we feel better about ourselves, we take more forthright action, make clearer decisions. Challenges are more easily overcome, obstacles more easily dissolved. That's *Raw Magic* in a nutshell; it's a win-win-win situation. Your body, your health, your mind, your life, your family, your friends, your planet; everyone's happier. It's a simple concept, but it really does have the power to change the world. It's time for us decide for ourselves that this is the future, and the future is now.

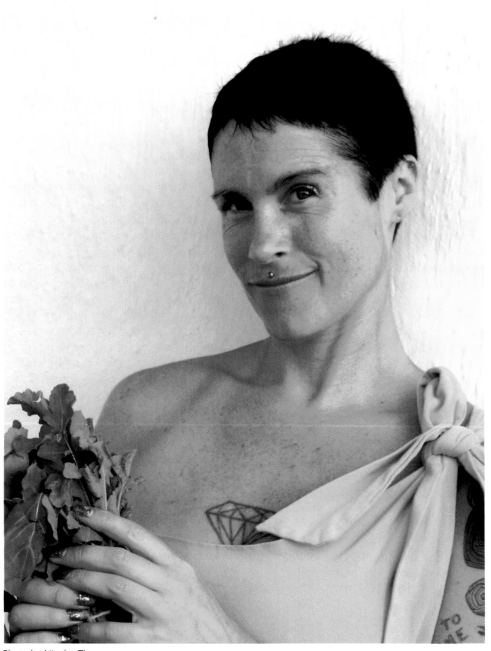

Photo by Nicolas Thorsen

Why Eat Raw Foods?

I made the conscious decision to "become a raw fooder" in 1993, and I can say, hand on heart, that every year it keeps getting better. For sure, there are challenges that arise in my life: I uncover emotional issues I need to work on; I encounter situations in my life that I need to change to move forward; more problems occur that demand a clear sharp focus to resolve; physical detoxification and healing comes up. But month on month, I find myself with increased levels of vitality. The joy I feel just through existing on this beautiful planet bubbles up and up; the energy and enthusiasm I have for life surges through my veins. The positivity and passion I feel for making the world a better place just keeps growing, no matter the setbacks I encounter on the way. I am more able to keep a clear intention and understand the steps I must take to reach my chosen goals. Every time I reach a new level of awareness and understanding, another one opens up before me. This journey is infinite, and it just keeps getting more magical.

I see raw foods as an integral part of optimum health and vitality. When you are eating pure plant foods with all their energy and life force intact, you are assisting your body in tuning into its own wisdom which is aligned with that of the earth from which the plants have grown. One of the basic tenets of raw foods is to eat food as close to the source as possible, sunfoods. So we don't generally eat animals and animal products, because the animals have gained their nourishment from the plants, and the plants are one step closer to receiving energy direct from the sun. Many of the superfoods grow in mountainous regions, e.g. maca, gojis—they are literally closer to the sun! Raw foods assist us in helping our bodies vibrate at the highest possible frequency; eating this way unlocks the potential within us to become more fully who we are.

Raw foods form the basis of a successful health program for a variety of reasons.

Enzymes

When we heat food above 42° C (118° F), the enzyme content is destroyed. Enzymes are necessary for almost every function in the body, especially digestion. As children, our bodies manufacture all the enzymes we need, but after adolescence we stop being able to make them ourselves and become dependent on food sources to get them. Enzymes are associated with aging; a diet high in enzymes promotes youthfulness and immortality! I consider them so important, I take extra enzyme supplementation with my raw food diet, which I find gives me even more energy and strengthens my immunity.

Nutritional Content

Nearly all foods have a higher nutritional content when eaten raw; heat destroys many vitamins, minerals, and amino acids. There are a few exceptions, such as lycopene, found in tomatoes and carrots. Lycopene can still be absorbed by the body if the cell walls have been broken down, by juicing for example.

Whole, Unprocessed

Generally, raw fooders eat foods that are less denatured. They are consuming less chemicals and artificial additives and preservatives with their foods. They are getting more fiber, and a higher water content.

Alkalinity

Thanks largely to the work of Dr. Robert O. Young, the public are becoming more widely aware of the benefits of a high alkaline diet. Most junk foods and heavily processed foods are acidic, causing a stress on the body which increases weight gain and decreases immunity. Ideally, the diet should be made up of at least 70% alkaline foods. A raw food diet high in vegetables easily satisfies this requirement. When our systems are alkalized, we feel calmer, can think more clearly, feel more on top of things, and have a stronger immune system.

Immune System

Cooked foods put a greater strain on the immune system than raw foods. When cooked foods are eaten, the body has an immune response known as leucocytosis. This does not occur when raw foods are eaten, although cooked foods can be eaten if they form less than 50% of the meal, and the raw foods are eaten first, in which case the body does not produce leucocytes. Generally, raw fooders find they are less prone to catching viruses than when they ate cooked foods, and when they do catch them, they tend to get them less severely and to shake them off faster.

Raw fooders tend to eat from four main food groups: vegetables, fruits, nuts and seeds, and sprouts (grains and pulses). From these foods, we can get all the requirements that conventional nutritionists state we need. To be successful, I believe a raw food diet should consist of at least 50% vegetables, the majority being green vegetables such as lettuce, spinach, rocket, broccoli, kale, celery, cucumber. The green leafy vegetables contain the most minerals and are also a surprisingly good source of protein. Juicing vegetables is an excellent way to up our daily intake. Fruit should be eaten minimally as a high fruit diet upsets blood sugar levels and can contribute to tooth decay. Try and eat local and seasonal fruit in preference to tropical fruits, which have lost a lot of their freshness and vitality as they have been shipped across the world. Nuts are a good source of protein but are generally acidic and mucus-forming. Soak nuts before using to activate enzyme inhibitors, and try and use seeds in preference. Seeds such as sesame, sunflower and pumpkin are highly nutritious, more easily digestible, and less acidic. Sprouted foods, like lentil, alfalfa, sunflower, wheat and buckwheat, are one of the best sources of nutrition because they are guaranteed fresh, raw, seasonal and locally grown! Sprouts have a superhigh nutritional content, and are cheap and easy to grow yourself.

My current thinking is that the ideal daily raw food diet should look something like this:

- 2–3 liters highest quality water available (this can include nut and seed milks, teas, and juices)
- Around 50% (in volume) of local, organic seasonal vegetables

And a balanced mix from the following food groups:

- Nuts and seeds
- Sprouts and indoor greens
- Sea vegetables
- Fruits
- Superfoods

I think it's crucial to include daily EFAs in the form of flax oil and hemp oil (at least 1 tablespoon), and fermented foods and drinks such as sauerkraut or kombucha are also extremely beneficial.

I believe for raw foods to become successfully integrated into our existing lifestyle, it is important not to get too fixated on our diets. Many people fail because they set themselves unattainable goals which they can't stick to, and then they feel that the raw food diet must not be for them. For it to be sustainable, it is far better to introduce raw foods gradually than rush at it headlong. Just increasing 50% of your diet to raw will reveal the benefits to you, especially when combined with daily consumption of superfoods. The rest will come in time. Raw is a journey not a destination; it is the key to a door but we must walk through the doorway unassisted, with no crutches. When being 100% raw becomes the goal, we are missing the point; if sticking to the diet is making us unhappy because we can't share food with friends, we are getting it wrong. Emotional health is just as important as physical health, and it is vital we keep that perspective: preparing and eating your food with love is just as beneficial as the quality of the food itself. When done properly, we shouldn't have to think about it; raw is there to enable us to live our lives more fully, to free up energy to enjoy ourselves, not to become another set of rules to be entrapped by. Raw foods open up a whole new paradigm within us, a world of unlimited life and abundance, where there is no death, just a continual rebirthing process. The potential for the transformation of humanity as more and more people open themselves up to this way of being is mind-blowing.

If you are interested in finding out more about raw food nutrition, and want some recipes to get you started, I go into more detail in my earlier books, *Eat Smart, Eat Raw* and *Raw Living*.

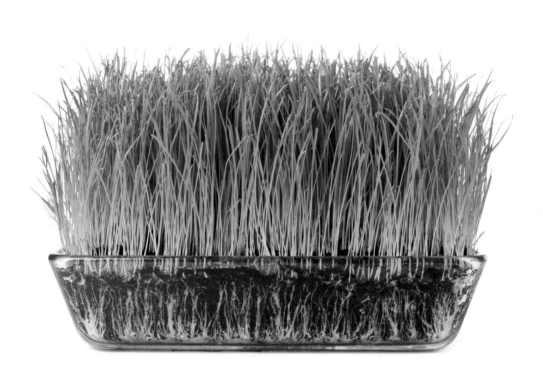

What Are Superfoods?

> "Be the change you wish to see in the world."
> —MAHATMA GANDHI

I adore superfoods. I have been eating them every day for over two decades, and I can say unequivocally that they provide me with that edge which helps me deal with the demands of life as a woman in the 21st century. Of course, I could do fine without them, but I don't want to just do fine, I don't want to just get by, I want to live a fulfilling and abundant life, and superfoods are a major factor in my being able to juggle and balance the varying and often contradictory elements of my world. I run a successful business, I enjoy many creative projects, I spend large amounts of quality time with my children, I have a full and fun social life, I am a conscientious and dedicated homemaker, and I get plenty of time in solitude to meditate and reflect. I am not leading a life that everyone isn't capable of, and I don't come from an exceptional background. I have had little support from family and society in my life because of the unconventional paths I have chosen to take, and I have lived for long periods of my life in relative poverty. But I had a dream, and I kept focused on that dream, and

my focus has led me to this point today. As a teenager growing up in the 1980s I knew there must be more to life than the picture of doom and gloom presented to us in the media, and the drudgery and boredom of my parents' lives. I sought to find alternatives, to find a deeper truth, a more beautiful way of living. My journey brought me back time and time again to the answer that all we have, all we need, is here in the moment, and the more we live life in our highest truth at every turn, the more we are rewarded. "Being the change" means being aligned in body and heart, constantly reminding ourselves of our focus and our truth in life, of how we can play our part to make the world a better place. And that is how I came to be so passionate about superfoods, foods that help create that inner and outer alignment in our lives.

People are becoming more familiar with the idea of superfoods, but there still remains a lot of confusion as to what actually qualifies as a superfood. I would classify them as natural plant foods which have two primary qualities: firstly, they are exceptionally high in nutrition and thereby provide the body with increased energy, and secondly, they have special intrinsic properties which can enhance our lives greatly. In my book, broccoli and blueberries are not superfoods! They may be excellent food choices, but they don't have the incredible charge and power of true superfoods. True superfoods really do make superbeings!

Because all the nutritional properties of these foods are so packed in, they are amazingly efficient, and make the body's job of extracting what it needs and utilizing it so much easier. When our bodies are getting their requirements met abundantly, and when the digestive process isn't being strained in the process, so much energy is released, we feel the revitalizing effects very quickly. This is a major factor in their growing popularity; the difference in your performance between when you take them and when you don't is remarkably obvious. Superfoods are in a different league from supplements because they are actually whole foods. Their natural synergy is preserved and the messages they send to the body are much more easy for it to receive and process than those of isolated components that have been manufactured in a laboratory.

As you are reading this book, you are very likely wondering why you haven't heard of many of these foods before. Most of them grow in areas where the land is purer and unspoiled because the indigenous populations are living lives of isolation and poverty, still relatively untouched by Western materialism. They are often celebrated and revered in their native countries, but unheard of outside of the regions where they are grown. As we Westerners start to realize the importance of really treating our bodies as temples, demand for innovative and original products increases, more research is done, and we are being introduced to many exciting new discoveries. As word spreads about their efficacy, people are joyfully consuming superfoods on a more and more regular basis.

If you are looking at the many superfood blends that are on the market, then I would advise you to remember that old adage "You get what you pay for." There is no such thing as a bad superfood, and I have never come across one which cannot help with healing to some degree, but the quality between brands varies immensely. Some are bulked out with cheaper fillers, others are of a higher potency. But what you are paying for when you buy these products is the formula development, the complicated manufacturing process of blending the powders to an exact recipe, the packaging and the branding. When you are taking the superfoods in this book, in my experience the body responds better because it is not being overwhelmed by the complex information contained in these branded blends. The body is like a child: it works best when it's being treated in as straightforward and uncomplicated a manner as possible, and is much happier being given one or two toys at a time to play with than a huge toy box where it's just going to lose half the pieces and then not be able to find the bit that it wants!

When you first enter the world of superfoods, it can be hard trying to decide which ones are right for you. They all have unique qualities which makes it hard to say that one is better or worse; it's like trying to compare peas and carrots or an apple with a banana. Some days, you fancy an apple, some days are banana days. It's best to start with just two or three, so you can notice their effects, and get to know them, then you can tune in and decide which ones you need at a particular time. It's also not easy recommending a daily dosage. It is always advisable to start off with a little and work up until you reach a level you feel comfortable with. Often the body will go through a healing crisis as it rebalances. Old complaints like skin problems or gut reactions may flare up, in which case return to a minimum maintenance dose, allow yourself some time to rest and let the body do its thing, and after a few days you should be feeling you've reached a new level of vitality as you've cleared your old stuff out.

Virtually all the superfoods in this book contain substances which regulate the body's metabolism and thus control cravings. They help us tune into the body's natural appetite, so that when you are eating superfoods on a daily basis, it becomes really hard to overeat or undereat. When superfoods are an integral part of your daily diet, you just don't get hungry in the same way. Low blood sugar, unhealthy food cravings, and issues around weight become a thing of the past. Weaknesses over food start to fade away, and sustained energy and vitality replace them. When I wrote *Eat Smart, Eat Raw*, one of my sayings was "If you want to lose weight, stop counting calories and start counting nutrients." Perhaps now we should change that to "Stop counting calories and start eating superfoods." Not only are weight issues a major factor in illness, they are a pre-occupying concern for so many people in society, particularly women. Think how much female power will be released when women stop obsessing over their dress size and are able to channel that trapped energy into more positive and creative pursuits!

It is the alchemy contained within these foods that puts them in the elite class of superfoods. It is an incredible nutritional profile, combined with an amazing vibration from the land where they are grown, and then presented within an easily accessible and bioavailable form that the body naturally recognizes and understands. Superfoods are "you can have your cake and eat it" foods, foods of enlightenment, foods of the gods. They fulfill both our needs from food: to be delicious, nurturing, irresistibly good, and satisfying, but also to meet all our nutritional requirements and fuel our bodies to the optimum. You need to love your food while you are eating it, and it needs to love you while it's in your body. It's all about the love, and double the love isn't just love plus love, it creates a magic which is infinite love. Eating these foods cause chemical reactions in your brain which put you on the right pathways, they guide you back to yourself, your inner wisdom, and enable you to make empowered choices which will create the life of your dreams. When we are living in accord with our higher intelligence, we become tuned in to ourselves and each other, and the magic flows. These foods nourish our bodies at the deepest level, the cellular level, and when we create harmony and alignment in our bodies, it manifests in our lives. That's why superfoods create superbeings. And the world really needs more superbeings right now.

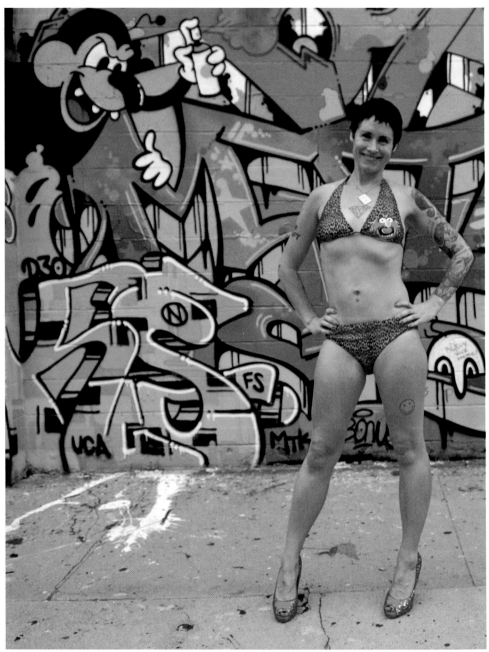

Photo by Phat Teddy

How To Have A Magic Day, Every Day

A fulfilling and healthy lifestyle needs to contain a balance of elements to keep you running on all levels. If you are too much in your head, on the computer all day, you're always going to be feeling a lack, that there is something missing in your life, because you're stuck in one place ignoring so much of the world around you. Likewise if you spend a lot of time doing things for other people and none on your own doing things for yourself, you're going to start feeling resentful and used. We find fulfillment through service, through giving, through knowing we have done our bit that day to make the world a better place. And we need to keep that in balance with the work we do on our own inner soul growth. Too much giving and we get burnt out; too much complacency and we are not contributing to the greater good. It demands skill to keep the balance between fulfilling our roles in the world and preserving our internal core, a skill which in itself needs working on and developing throughout our lives. I believe there are five elements we need to include in our daily routines to keep whole, to keep dancing. Of course we rarely get to include them all every day, but if we make them our focus, if we keep them in balance within the week, then everything else flows around that.

1. Exercise is integral to a healthy body, oxygenating the blood and stimulating the lymph. Daily stretching helps to relieve tension and improve mental clarity, loosening mental as well as physical rigidity.
2. Love makes the world go 'round. Human beings need love to flourish as much as we need food and water. Spending time with people you treasure and who treasure you is the most important part of your day.
3. Service. What is your gift? Your unique individual special talent that no one else has. What do you love to do to make other people happy? This is your life's work, your mission on the planet, and is usually manifold.
4. Food of love is the biggest gift we can give ourselves. Feed yourself the best organic, seasonal, local produce available, and see the world offer you the best right back at you.
5. Meditation. Time spent alone is essential for inner peace. Even if you can only find ten minutes early in the morning, that is time well spent to set your focus and intent for the day.

I have friends who are healers, singers and mothers; artists, musicians and fathers; managers, writers and chefs. Many combine something in the healing arts with something creatively expressive; many combine something more left-brain like teaching with something more right-brain like design; the vast majority do not have a "boss" but work independently. In virtually every case, what we do benefits those around us *at the same time as* enriching our own lives. As we come into our power, we discover these different strands to ourselves, and it becomes our passion to share these with the world. This is what we mean when we call ourselves multidimensional beings: people who are experiencing life in all its different facets, who enjoy a rich and rewarding social life, family life, love life, work life, and creative life, and who successfully dance between the different, often paradoxical aspects of themselves, by retaining a deep connection to their divinity.

The key to a happy life is simplicity and sustainability. If we are all living in tune with the environment and in harmony with our fellow beings, if we are not plundering the earth's resources and abusing her abundance, then our needs can be met effortlessly. All the most effective tools for living are simple, easy and often free. As we come together with the same vision, we develop communities which operate harmoniously and make life even easier as we share the burdens and responsibilities of day-to-day life. We live in simple and sustainable dwellings, and we grow our food simply and sustainably; we spend our time in pursuits that give back to the earth rather than benefiting man at the earth's expense; we use natural household and bodycare products, and clothes, bedding and towels made of fabrics like hemp and organic cotton. We don't need endless possessions because we have inner peace, we don't consume more than is necessary because we have inner contentment. We don't pollute the water and the land with chemicals. This is the paradise vision: it is easy to achieve, simple to manifest, once it becomes the consensus reality. Playing in Gaia's garden, nurturing and being nurtured, healing the planet with our love, one day at a time, one acre at a time. It's not an impossible dream; there are communities dotted all over the world already living this way, and the more of us who move toward this vision, the more possible it becomes.

When we are flowing with the universe, the universe looks after us. When we are living in our most spiritual truth, vibrating at our highest level, magic occurs and miracles manifest. Our needs are met, we are provided for, our dreams start to come true. Synchronicities abound, joy overflows, love is everywhere. All it takes is that leap of imagination, to step out of the box, to take risks with the unknown, to not be scared of not understanding and not being in control. It just means taking small steps every day, moment by moment, and before you know it, you have the best life ever.

How To Get Your B12

This is one of the most common questions I get asked. Where do you get your B12 from? Do you take supplements? Yes, it is one of the few vitamins that is next to impossible to find on a raw vegan diet. There are many rational answers I can give to that question, facts and statistics I can trot out. I have looked into the subject, and it is not something I worry about. If you want to know more, I would refer you to the work of Gabriel Cousens who is very knowledgeable on the subject, and whose opinion I respect greatly. What does concern me, and what I believe is more valuable to share with you, is how to get your cosmic B12. Here are 12 ways to find your Bliss.

1. Everything happens for a reason.

There is a divine intelligence at work in the universe that is orchestrating a whole grand masterplan. We cannot expect to comprehend its workings, that's why it's a higher intelligence. When we hand over that control and understand we are just actors on a stage, that brings with it a huge sense of relief and inner peace. The more that you hand the power over, the more the universe looks after you, and the more you can enjoy being in the moment.

2. I am doing exactly what the universe wants me to do right here and now.

Find the perfection in the moment—it is always present, it's just that we cannot always see it. But know that you are right where you are meant to be, doing what you are meant to be doing, at every instant.

3. My job is to be a clear channel for my higher self to work through.

All we need to do is access the divine intelligence which exists in each and every one of us, encoded in our cells, our DNA. We also hold programming, patterns both inherited and learned, which blocks the messages of our DNA. So it is a perpetual dance between working on clearing the channels, and manifesting the intentions of our higher selves.

4. All that matters is the moment.

The whole of reality exists right in the here and now. It always was and it always will be. All that matters is being in the moment and accessing the divine within it. If you think what you're doing in the 3-D is important, or that you understand, or that you're in control, you're on the wrong track. Truth is a magical mystery beyond our present state of understanding.

5. Love it all.
Everything that happens to me is a manifestation of my own holographic matrix; outer reality is simply a reflection of my own inner state of being. So all I see is a part of me, and the best way to deal with anything that troubles us is to love it into submission. Love dissolves all patterns.

6. It's all an illusion.
The material world is an illusion, a thinly disguised veil for multidimensional reality. It's a game, and it's our mission to see through the veil, penetrate the illusion, and reveal the hidden truths within the matrix.

7. Money and time are tools utilized by the dark forces to keep us submissive.
Money is not real; it's the biggest illusion of them all and everyone buys into it. The universe is abundant, and if we are serving her, then she will take care of us. Time is only a linear representation of a point in an infinite universe and as such is pretty meaningless way of plotting change and growth. Being always present in the moment you enter the bliss of the eternal now.

8. All darkness comes from a sense of separation.
There is no separation, only oneness; separation is illusion; we are never alone. Find the unity and the oneness and dissolve the darkness, the fear, anger, resentment and lack.

9. There are beings from other dimensions looking out for us.
We are far from being the only intelligent life force in the universe. Angels, archangels, ascended masters, members of the Galactic Federation are all around us, guiding us, nurturing us, loving us.

10. Humanity is going through a shift in consciousness.
We are at the dawn of a new golden age, ascension, enlightenment, even the second coming or the end of the world! There are many different ways to interpret it, all of them inadequate for the full multidimensional glory that we are just beginning to get glimpses of.

11. We find fulfillment in service.
The more we walk our truth and help guide humanity into the light, the more fulfilling a life we lead. The more we give, the more bliss we receive. Balance that with your own inner work to find perfection in your life.

12. The universe loves me and it wants me to be happy.
Whenever you feel troubled and challenged, just repeat this mantra. It's not going to be hard this time, it's going to be easy. The universe loves me and it wants me to be happy.

The Left Brain/Right Brain Dichotomy

It is scientifically established that the two hemispheres of the brain have different functions. The left hemisphere is responsible for tasks we think of as more male-oriented: linear, rational, logical thought. The left brain is the I, the independent thinker, the ego, which understands itself as separate from the rest of the world, an isolated part. This is where our competitive instinct comes from, as we feel we must fight for self-preservation; it is also where we feel fear and anger. The right brain is the more feminine aspect of the mind; the creative, nurturing, giving aspect. The right brain has no sense of self, ego or separation, it experiences the self only as part of the greater whole, in oneness and union. The right brain has no understanding of time, it occupies the infinite moment. The right brain is the genius inside all of us, a unique spark of creativity that has something unrivaled and extraordinary to offer to the world.

Western culture is left-brain dominant. Some of us may have developed our right hemispheres more than others, but all of us are ruled by the left brain, the notions of time and the fight for self-preservation being controlling factors in our lives. Tony Wright, an English raw fooder and consciousness researcher, has a theory that it was not always like this, that what is biblically known as the Fall was the point when man left paradise and became left-brain dominant. In order to achieve enlightenment, to recover our natural state of bliss and return earth to the paradise garden it once was, we must learn to balance the two hemispheres.

It is a startlingly simple concept, and one into which all paradigms fall. It doesn't matter which religion, which psychoanalytical theory, which social or scientific model you look at, they all fit into this one simple paradigm. All the ills in the world can be whittled down to one cause: the repression of the right brain by the left.

I believe that raw foods stimulate the right brain; superfoods fire up the right brain, especially cacao. Meditation, yoga, chanting, and all creative and artistic pursuits, all help build new pathways in the brain which create a greater state of balance. As we move more into our right brains, we literally learn new ways of thinking. We begin to consider what is good for the whole in a given situation, not what will purely benefit ourselves. We operate less from a place of fear, poverty and scarcity, and more from a place of love, trust and abundance. Because we are tuning in to the universal mind or infinite being, synchronicities abound, and time and again things miraculously fall into place at the last moment. We are in the flow, and the flow is strong in us.

In my experience, eating superfoods is the surest and easiest way to build up the right brain and create new pathways. Cacao is the major way to do this, especially in combination with other superfoods containing rare trace minerals like Etherium Gold and Blue Manna. The longer we consume these foods on a daily basis, the more we open up to our inner worlds (the right brain), and are less constrained by society's expectations of us, our left-brain programming.

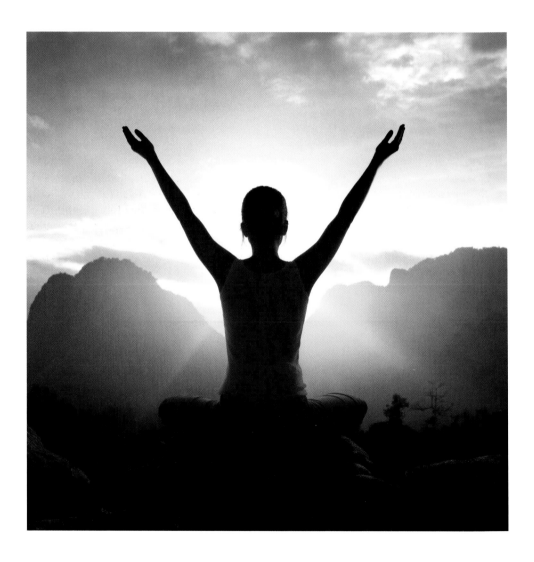

Cacao

"I could give up chocolate, but I'm not a quitter."
—ANONYMOUS

"Anything is good, if it's covered in chocolate."
—JO BRAND, COMEDIENNE

The cacao bean comes from the cacao fruit, which is a pod growing mainly in Africa and South America, similar to a papaya. The fruit is delicious, and consumed by the native people, white and creamy and not overly sweet; similar to custard apple. Each fruit contains between 20–50 beans, and the cacao bean is what all chocolate is made from. So why have we only recently discovered the health benefits of chocolate? The average bar of chocolate you find on the supermarket shelves is made from cocoa solids. Fermenting the beans, then drying them out, makes cocoa solids. The beans are then cleaned and roasted, and this heating process destroys many of their nutritional properties. The roasted beans then have their shells removed and the result are the nibs, broken-up bits of bean. The nibs are then intensely heated again, so the oils melt to form what is known as chocolate liquor. The chocolatiers take the cocoa solids and at very high temperatures, mix them with ingredients—usually milk, sugar and emulsifiers—to make a chocolate bar. So the cacao bean goes through three heating processes, has many of its beneficial oils removed, is combined with foods that are not optimally healthy, and the chocolate that we experience is but a poor shadow of the real thing. In Europe, regulations state that to be called milk chocolate, a bar must contain at least 10% cocoa solids—so in a high street chocolate bar, only one-tenth of the actual ingredients have to be this denatured form of chocolate, and the rest is fattening, bad for your teeth, acidic, and unbalancing for the blood sugar! The discovery of the raw cacao bean is analogous to having only been fed white sliced bread our whole lives and suddenly discovering the power of the whole wheat grain; or only drinking orange juice made from concentrate out of a carton and having freshly squeezed for the first time. Despite this, it is still one of the most popular foods on the planet. There is no other food which people become so openly and willingly addicted to! This gives us some idea of the power of cacao.

Pottery evidence of the use of cacao dates back to Honduras in 2000 B.C., although the human use of cacao fruit may go back as far as 15,000 years. It originates from South America, and the first civilization that is considered to have cultivated cacao was the Olmecs of Mexico. The Mayans learned about cacao from the Olmecs and made it a central part of their civilization. There is much archaeological evidence of pottery and wall carvings, some of their rulers were named after cacao, and they even had cacao gods. As well as imbibing cacao, they used it in coming-of-age rituals and as a sacred offering in religious ceremonies. The Aztec civilization followed that of the Mayans, and they too conferred great prestige on the cacao pod. The beans were so revered by the Mayans and Aztecs that they used them as currency. In the Aztec city of Texcoco, the city budget was as much as 32,000 beans a day! One fish was worth three cacao beans, one avocado was worth one cacao bean, a canoe was one hundred beans. Incredibly, they continued to be used as currency in Mexico until 1887. It was the Spanish explorer Hernan Cortes, who conquered Mexico in the sixteenth century, who brought cacao to Europe. Cortes described cacao as "the divine drink which builds up resistance and fights fatigue. A cup of this precious drink permits a man to walk for a whole day without food." Christopher Columbus also recorded coming across it on his travels. Carl von Linnaeus, the eighteenth-century Swedish scientist, gave the tree its Latin name, *theobroma cacao*, "cacao, the food of the gods." Now, over two-thirds of the world's cacao is grown in Africa, mainly on the Cote d'Ivoire.

In its raw, untampered-with state, the cacao bean is one of the most nutrient-dense foods known to man. It contains over 300 chemical compounds, making it one of the most complex and nutritionally significant foods available to us. It is a premium source of minerals, vitamins, antioxidants, protein and healthy fats.

Minerals

Cacao is one of the very best known dietary sources of magnesium and sulphur. Magnesium is an essential mineral in which most of us are deficient. Like calcium, it is important for building strong bones, and assists in converting EFAs in the body. It provides essential support for the heart, helps relieve premenstrual tension, and is a natural laxative. It is an excellent source of sulphur, known as the beauty mineral because it is so beneficial for the hair, eyes, skin and teeth. Cacao also contains significant amounts of iron, phosphorous, and the B vitamin group.

Antioxidants

Cacao contains 10% antioxidant flavonols, nearly twice the amount found in red wine and three times that found in green tea. The antioxidants in cacao are easily absorbable by the body, and have been shown to assist in cardiovascular health, and help prevent against cancer.

The ORAC score is the official U.S. measurement for antioxidant levels in food. The ORAC score for raw cacao powder is virtually off the scale—995 units per gram, at least seven times more than that of normal dark chocolate.

Neurotransmitters

Neurotransmitters are chemicals which transmit nerve impulses across a synapse, i.e. they effect chemical reactions in the brain. Cacao is home to the neurotransmitter anandamide, known as "the bliss chemical," an endogenous cannabinoid naturally found in the human brain. Cacao is the only food other than cannabis to contain cannabinoids. Cacao also contains anandamide inhibitors, which means that our bodies' abilities to break down anandamide is decreased, and so the blissed-out feeling lasts longer. Cacao also contains significant amounts of tryptophan, an essential amino acid which the brain uses to make the neurotransmitter serotonin. Serotonin is known for the feelings of euphoria it creates; the dance-drug Ecstacy causes large amounts of serotonin to be released in the brain.

Phenylethylamine

PEA is known as "the molecule of joy," and only present in two foods, chocolate and blue-green algae. It is the chemical produced in the brain when we are fully happy and immersed in the moment, especially when involved in a creative act like writing or painting, dancing or making music. PEA is also very good for the brain, and improves brain function. When I take the PEA extract Blue Manna, I feel more focused, alert and intelligent. Physically, it promotes healthy joints and tis-

sues. And if all that wasn't enough, PEA also affects the neurotransmitters dopamine and norepinephrine, which increase mental positivity. It is the presence of PEA which largely seems to account for the common folklore wisdom that chocolate makes a good substitution for sex, as we get the same increased levels of PEA when we are in love. "Some 50% of women reportedly claim to prefer chocolate to sex, though this response may depend on the attributes of the interviewer." (chocolate.org)

Aphrodisiacs

A box of chocolates is the most popular gift to give on Valentine's day. As well as the loved-up feelings we get from the PEA in chocolate, the neurotransmitters affected by chocolate make us feel happy and alert, and the minerals magnesium and sulphur both loosen the muscles and make us more relaxed. On top of that, cacao is one of the best dietary sources of arginine, an amino acid also known as nature's Viagra. Arginine increases blood flow to the heart and the genitals, increasing arousal and improving sexual appetite.

MAO Inhibitors

Cacao contains monoamine oxidase inhibitors (MAOIs) which inhibit monoamine oxidase enzymes (MAOs). This has the effect of increasing the levels of neurotransmitters in the body, and having an antidepressant effect. When we are young, we naturally produce high levels of neurotransmitters, thus MAOIs facilitate a youthful attitude to life and have anti-aging properties. They also act as an appetite suppressant. Cacao seems to have the effect of regulating the body's natural appetite: it helps us tune into what our bodies actually need, rather than eating out of habit or for emotional comfort. Most regular consumers of raw cacao report weight loss and an improved ability to stabilize their weight at the level they feel most comfortable with. Additionally, MAOIs are present in significant amounts in shamanistic plants such as ayahuasca. This would account for the enhanced psychic sensibility that many cacao-lovers experience.

Stimulants

Cacao contains subtle amounts of the methylxanthines caffeine and theobromine. These are both stimulants, however both are proving to have far different effects when consumed raw rather than cooked. The presence of caffeine is one of the primary reasons people cite for avoiding chocolate, but in our experience, the caffeine in raw chocolate has little to no effect. Personally, I have a highly developed and sensitive system which cannot tolerate even small doses of substances such as alcohol and caffeine. Before we discovered raw chocolate, if I was to eat even the tiniest amount of cooked vegan dark chocolate, I would feel the negative effects of the caffeine. I get a tense, wired, edgy feeling from caffeine that I never get from raw cacao. When we first started making chocolate bars, one batch of cacao nibs we were sent had been toasted by accident. It only took a few days of consuming these toasted nibs for us all to notice an increase in aggressive feelings and mood swings. This to me was enough proof that the caffeine in cacao only has negative effects once it has been heated. Homeopathic research

has come to a similar conclusion that the physiological changes are caused by substances released during heating.

So why is cacao such a magical food? Why do people go completely crazy for it, while others are vehemently against it? I believe cacao is a wake-up food. It wakes you up to your full power, to who you truly are, to the potentiality of the moment, to the infinite and abundant nature of the universe. For a lot of people, this is too much to handle. We are brought up to believe in limitation and suffering. For people whose whole lives are based around this paradigm, cacao brings up too much fear. How could I step outside of the box I've created for myself? How could I let go of my ego's definition of who I am, and be fully, spiritually in the moment? For many people this is too big a leap to make, and they cannot find a place for the cacao gods in their hearts. But for the majority of people, the opposite is true. Most people feel limited and restricted in their lives. They are dying to break out of the box, to live a bit more freely, to embrace who they fully are and be given a chance to soar. Cacao gives them a taste of what this could be like, and that is a wonderful feeling. And remember, with our thoughts we create the world. So when we experience that cacao high, every time we break out of a restricting thought pattern, we are telling the universe we are willing to accept a greater truth, a higher reality.

For example, you are having a tough morning with the kids. Two of them are fighting, and the baby has had you awake all night. There is a big pile of washing to do, and a heap of emails you are dying to get a peek at. It's 11 a.m. and you are starting to flag. Eat a piece of toast, or a few rice cakes, and you are more likely to stay locked in that negative pattern. How hard this all is; why do mums get so dumped on; why don't I have more help? But eat some raw cacao with its super-dynamic loved-up switched-on energy, and your whole mindset changes. You find yourself laughing at their bickering instead of taking it seriously, and rather than shouting at them and losing your temper, you join in the rough and tumble and make a game of it. Or you notice what a glorious sunny day it is outside and bundle them all up to the swings where you bump into one of your favorite friends and sit there putting the world to rights while the children get to burn off their energy. The vibration you are sending out to the universe then is that parenting is fun and easy, and miraculously the universe sends you situations that match that vibration; your husband comes home and spontaneously attacks the wash basket for you instead of watching TV, and a friend offers to have the kids over the next day which gives you a chance to disappear into your emails. Whereas if you had been in a grump all day about the hopelessness of your situation and the misery of parenthood, that is just the situation the universe delivers for you, the next day, and the next day, and the next day, until you can change that record in your head.

Cacao is the food of the goddess. Goddess energy is about being in the moment; it is about surrender, acceptance, and loving everything. It is about flowing, and being present and giving, giving, and more giving. When we eat

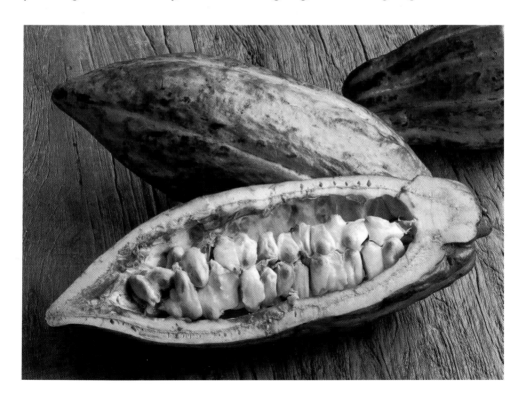

cacao, it puts us right back in touch with our goddess energy. It puts us fully in the moment, and loving it, ready to give some more. For instance, you have had a long busy day at work. You've come straight home for dinner and had a delicious raw soup. You know you should call your mum because she called over the weekend and you haven't had a chance to return her call; she will be waiting, getting anxious that you are neglecting her. Have some ice cream for dessert and you'll more likely end up in front of the TV, feeling guilty that you haven't called again. But eat a piece of chocolate as an after-dinner treat, and bam! There is that extra energy you needed to pick up the phone and show your mum you really do care. You speak for half an hour, and she feels so much better because she got to speak with you, and you feel so much better because you made your mum happy.

Cacao is also a major sunfood. Sunfoods are the foods that carry strong yang energy: they are expansive, they help us reach up and out and are strengthening and energizing. They keep our energy rising and ascending. Thus they help us deal with our blockages, because they give us the insight to rise above them, to meet them head on and to move beyond them. Perhaps there is a boy that you like. He said he would call that evening, but he has a habit of letting you down. When he does call, he is always charming and funny and gorgeous; unfortunately, he more often doesn't call than he does. Instead of sitting at home, wasting time on Facebook, waiting for the phone to ring, you eat some raw chocolate, call up a girlfriend, and go out for a dance. And who knows, maybe you meet a charming, funny, gorgeous boy who does call!

Are you getting the picture now? At first sight, it may seem simplistic to say that a food can change your life. But what we are really saying is your consciousness creates your reality, with your thoughts you make the world. Basically put, we are all a chain of chemical reactions, endless cause and effect. The food you put in your mouth is made of many chemicals; these have an effect on your body and consciousness; which then has an effect on how you react to any given situation; which then has a knock-on effect on the rest of your day, your week, your life, and also the lives of everyone you come into contact with. Cacao is made of over 300 chemical constituents; it is one of the most complex foods known to man. It melts at body temperature, so when you put it in your mouth, all those chemicals explode as they hit the tongue. So it is such an all-encompassing, expansive, abundant food, that that is how you feel when you eat it; at its best, it gives you the ability to feel that you could deal with any situation that arises in the next moment; it makes you feel god-like, a superbeing. This is what we mean when we talk about superbeings: people who are so in their flow, so in tune with their higher purpose, so aligned with their inner truth, that they are not afraid of living in their full power, they know they can deal with whatever life throws at them. And precisely because they are so positive, so visionary, so fearless, they attract in less and less situations of stress, doubt, negativity and poverty, and instead create a reality about them that is blissful, assured and abundant.

Another magical property of cacao is the way it acts as a platform for other foods. It has a synergistic effect on the ingredients that you mix it with that increases their effect exponentially. For that reason, I often put a little cacao in with my other superfoods. You don't need a lot, just half a teaspoon of powder or a teaspoon of nibs, but it gives them a lift, an extra edge. Instead of just taking maca straight, mix a little chocolate in and the effects will be maca to the power of maca, maca squared. It's like cacao raises the vibration of whatever it comes into contact with, it shines a spotlight on it and allows it be fully who it is, it brings out the very best qualities of a food. Naturally, this works in reverse as well; a tablespoon of maca or a teaspoon of suma in your chocolate rounds out the cacao experience, brings an extra depth to the cacao magic, enhances the alchemy.

Many religions teach that the road to enlightenment is through a balance of the opposing forces within us. Life as we know it is about duality, and what propels us on is the searching for a resolution within that dynamic, a striving to find the unity, bliss and oneness behind it all. It is a perpetual dance between yin and yang, the dark and the light, heaven and earth. The more we learn to combine those energies, to allow them to co-exist within us, the closer we get to reaching nirvana. Cacao is the food of enlightenment because it is a sunfood (yang) and it is also the food of the goddess (yin). It brings together the two polarities within us. How does it do this? Culturally, we are taught to think of foods as either good for us and boring, or bad for us and fun; "you can't have your cake and eat it." When I was a child, eaters were divided into two clear-cut categories: the sanctimonious, weird and dull people who ate brown rice and lentils, or the life-affirming brigade who embraced everything and drank, smoked and ate dead animals. Gradually, over the decades, those stereotypes started to dissolve as the do-gooders realized they had to acknowledge their dark side, they couldn't abstain forever unless they really did want to be miserable; and the omnivores started to get sick in ever-increasing numbers. Cacao dissolves all those stereotypes completely. Here is the richest, darkest, most delicious, decadent, luxurious, divine-tasting food ever, and it also happens to be one of the number one dietary sources of minerals and antioxidants on the planet. One slice of one of my chocolate cakes has more nutrition in it than what most people would consider a healthy meal, something like stir-fry and noodles. When eaten on a regular basis, cacao really does blow your mind, because it blasts all your preconceptions of what is good and bad out of the window. It allows you to live beyond duality, to dance in the one. You can discover your darkness and live in your light all at the same time. It is the mother and the father energy all rolled into one; it nurtures you and comforts you, then it kicks you out the door and tells you to get the hell on with it.

What else? Yes, there's more, there's always more. Because cacao is the food of abundance. It helps us to experience the universe as infinite and eternal; it opens us up to the sense that we can keep flowing, keep living, keep loving. Life stops being a series of deaths and rebirths, and turns into a continual ecstatic "Yes!"

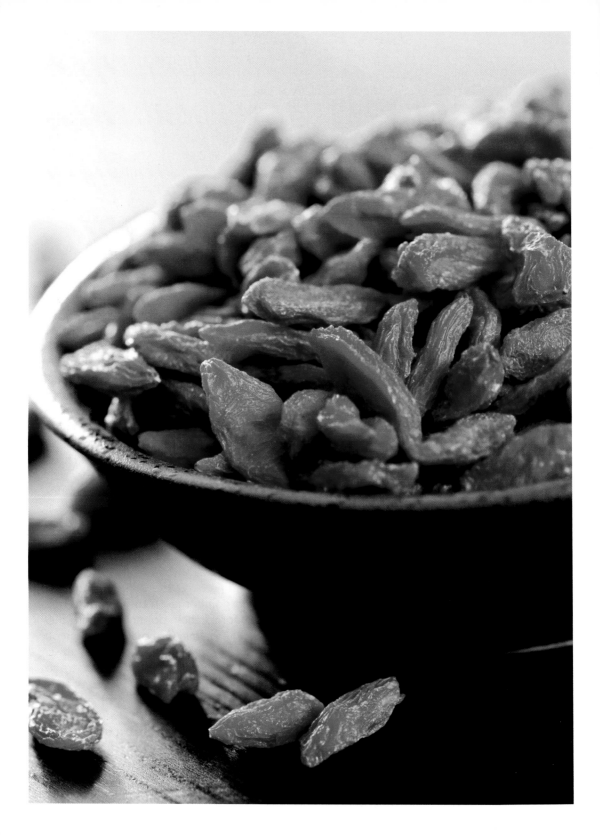

Gojis

In the UK, 2006 was the year of the goji berry.

It became the latest fad trend, mentioned in the same breath as a list of skinny A-list celebrities, flying off the shelves of Fresh & Wild, the subject of BBC News articles. So is there anything behind the hype? Are goji berries just overpriced raisins? The Chinese have been eating gojis for over 2,000 years, and are mildly amused at our sudden "discovery" of what is to them an everyday food. The Chinese consume gojis in many forms: they add them to rice and meat when cooking, they make them into wine, and they are a popular tea. In the West, they are more commonly consumed as a snack, either on their own or in bars and trail mixes, or in the form of juice (although most products marketed as goji juice actually have a very low goji content). Like tomatoes, peppers and potatoes, they are a member of the nightshade family. I often substitute them for dried tomatoes in savory recipes as they have a similar intense, vivid flavor. They can easily be found in Chinese herbalists as well as health food shops, although the quality is variable. Generally, the more bright orange in color gojis are the more likely they are to have been sprayed with high levels of pesticides—the deeper red, the better.

The berries grow on shrubs, and those that grow in the Chinese Ningxia region are said to be very high quality. Here they grow along the floodplains of the Yellow River, renowned for its mineral-rich silt. This is likely to be why goji berries are said to contain monatomic trace elements and be high in ormus energy (see p. 67): they are grown in ancient, mineral-rich soil. So great is the popularity of gojis, and their contribution to the economy, that in Ningxia they hold an annual goji berry festival. The berries must be harvested carefully, and cannot be touched because that will cause them to oxidize and turn black. They are picked by hand, by shaking them off the bushes and onto mats where they are sun-dried or taken to factories for dehydrating.

Admittedly, there is some hype around goji berries in the West. In their dried form, they do not contain 500 times the vitamin C of oranges—fresh off the bush, maybe, but as anyone knows, vitamin C is very sensitive to heat and light and easily destroyed. Although they contain antioxidants that are known to prevent aging, it is unlikely that there are Chinese people who lived to be over 200 years old by eating them. Eating goji berries alone will not make you lose weight, although as part of a healthy diet they will fulfill your nutritional requirements and help you tune into your body's natural appetite. But like all the superfoods in this book, they have a strong nutritional profile that assists the body in many different ways. And they also have that magical energetic quality, a "je ne sais quoi" which makes them uniquely irresistible. The Chinese say the only side effect of eating goji berries is laughing too much! I believe their popularity is largely down to the "have your cake and eat it" factor. Like cacao, gojis are fun. They taste like yummy little sweets, and you want to eat them, there is no element of chore or duty involved. But at the same time you are feeding your body one of the most nutrient-dense fruits on the planet, and giving yourself high doses of many vitamins, minerals and amino acids that you might be lacking.

In TCM (traditional Chinese medicine), goji berries are a yin food. They assist the liver and kidneys, enhance the immune system, and improve eyesight. Like ginseng, they are a tonic fruit, and nourish the heart and the internal organs. They are a valuable protein source, containing 18 of the 22 amino acids, including all eight essential amino acids, which makes them a great food for vegans, vegetarians, and developing children. They contain 22 minerals and trace minerals, thanks to the quality of the soil they are grown in. They are one of the best plant sources of iron and selenium, as well as containing significant amounts of calcium, potassium, and zinc. They are rich in vitamins, particularly the B group of vitamins, and exceptionally high in beta-carotene—more than carrots or apricots. It is the presence of carotenoids that gives them their reputation for improving eyesight. They are widely recognized for the amounts of polysaccharides they contain, which boost the immune system and reduce the risk of cancer. It is this combination of carotenoids and polysaccharides that make them such a valuable source of antioxidants. Contained in the seeds of the berries are significant amounts of omega-3 and omega-6 oils, the essential fatty acids.

Goji berries are associated with love, because of their bright red color, and the positive effect they have on the libido. Like cacao, they are a heart-centered food, so adding a few of them to any meal can help carry the qualities of all the other foods into our hearts. I wouldn't say goji berries are particularly energizing in the same way that, for example, maca or pollen are. But they do provide us with a certain vitality, a ray of energy that no other foods provide. Because they are grown in one of the purest places on earth, the Himalayan mountains, they have a pure, high vibration that uplifts us, which is why they are known as the "happy berry." It is this combination of being uplifting energetically and nourishing physically that makes them such a potent food. This humble little berry has the ability to simply add a little sunshine into your day (which is probably why they've caught on so much in the UK).

Maca

If I were the British Prime Minister, I would put maca on the NHS for everyone.

Only it wouldn't be the National Health Service, it would be the Nation of Happy Superfooders. Maca is an adaptogen, so it assists the body in restoring balance; whatever your health problem, whatever stresses you are under, maca will support your body in correcting any imbalances. It has also been demonstrated to regulate hormones, so is particularly beneficial for women. I very rarely meet anyone who has not felt a tangible improvement in their well-being from taking maca. And unlike taking a supplement like iron drinks, or calcium tablets, where you are not really sure if you are noticing the benefits, everyone feels maca instantly. Almost immediately, users report increased energy levels and improved stamina.

Maca is a root vegetable, from the same family of cruciferous vegetables as broccoli and cauliflower. It looks a little like a very large radish, and is used in food preparation in the same way as other starchy root vegetables such as parsnips and potatoes: boiled and mashed,

baked or fried. It is native to Peru, where it grows high in the Andes Mountains. The history of maca is a fascinating tale. In 1989, it was declared one of the "lost crops of the Incas," and the plant was in danger of extinction. But over the past couple of decades, interest in this amazing crop has grown in America, Europe and Japan, primarily for its effects on the libido, but also as a natural alternative to steroids for athletes, and a natural alternative to HRT for women. In 1979, there were only 25 cultivated hectares of maca in Peru; now there are over 2,000. This is a very good thing for the native people of Peru, whose communities are benefiting from job creation, increased cash flow, and recognition for their culture; not just from the growth in the maca industry, but other native crops such as lucuma, yacon, and cacao. On the whole, these crops are being traded fairly, with respect for the indigenous population. Peru is one of the poorest countries in the world, and their land is notoriously inhospitable. The Peruvian government is very protective of its native species, and will not allow the seeds to be exported, so that they can maintain the monopoly on their precious assets. Only the powders or extracts are allowed to be exported. That is why you never see whole maca root (or yacon or lucuma) outside of South America.

Maca has been popular among the indigenous peoples of Peru for as long as five thousand years. The Incans valued it so highly, they only permitted its use in the royal courts. When the Spanish conquistadors came to Peru in the sixteenth century, they were close to leaving, worn down by the harsh living conditions and their declining fertility levels. It was the discovery of maca that enabled them to stay in Peru, and they would trade in maca in preference to gold. Like cacao, maca has strong associates with gold energy, the ray that lifts us up to the sun, creates inner fire, auric expansion, and vibrational ascension.

Maca is one of the most powerful of the superfoods, so consequently you have to be very careful with it initially and use it with respect. It can have strong rebalancing and detoxifying effects. For instance, say you suffer badly from premenstrual tension every month. For your first cycle of taking maca, your PMS is likely to be more severe than ever. But by the second cycle, it should start to balance out, and by the third or fourth cycle will be disappearing completely. Or perhaps you suffer from chronic fatigue syndrome. After a few days of taking maca, you might start to feel more tired and wiped out than ever. But stick with it, and within a week those symptoms will pass, your energy levels will start to rebuild, and gradually you will recover a sustained energy and drive. I always advise people to start off with half a teaspoon of maca. If after three or four days that doesn't seem a lot, and you aren't noticing any effects, or conversely if it tastes

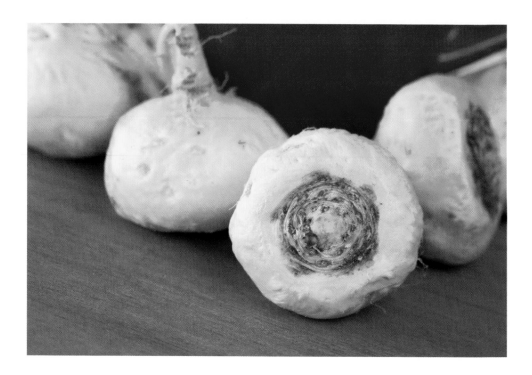

wonderful to you and you are craving more, then up the dose to a teaspoon. Keep upping it by half a teaspoon every three or four days until you reach your threshold. By this I mean the point at which you feel you have as much energy as you can cope with, and your detox symptoms start to reveal themselves. At this point, you might want to lower the dose again, although it is important not to stop taking it completely if you want its magic to work. Once your detox has passed, and you have flushed out the imbalances you can take as much maca as you like. Remember, it is just a vegetable. In Peru, they eat it like we eat potatoes; they fry it and serve it as chips with chili sauce at roadside stalls, or they mash it and make a kind of porridge with it. They also enjoy it as an alcoholic beverage, making beers, liqueurs, and cocktails with it. Once your body has readjusted itself, you do not need to limit the amounts you are taking; I take up to two tablespoons a day.

Maca is the plant that grows at the highest altitudes in the world, nine to eleven thousand feet above sea level; there is no other plant that grows in such inhospitable terrain. For this reason, it gives us that energy to climb that mountain: if life seems like an uphill struggle to you, if you can't see how you can reach your goals, the peak of your personal mountain, maca will provide you with that inner fire and insight to keep on going. The maca plant has a very high frost tolerance, so it gives you the strength to battle against the cold. I am known amongst my friends for having little sensitivity to the cold, and refusing to put the central heating on in winter! I am sure this is due in part to the large

amounts of maca in my diet, as well as the long time I have been raw. It's not that I don't notice the cold, it's just that it doesn't bother me, it doesn't disturb my internal balance. In fact, maca grows under a variety of extreme conditions: frost, intensive sunlight and high winds. Hence it gives us that really sturdy, invincible energy.

Truly, maca provides one of the best sources of energy I have ever come across. It is instant and long-lasting. It makes me feel strong and grounded, calm and in control, not wild and over-excited like too much chocolate can! Pollen is a brilliant source of energy too, but it is high in sugar and too much can affect blood glucose levels. Because maca is a root vegetable, the energy it provides is much steadier. It is a natural partner to cacao, and also goes very well with oats, which provide the same sort of slow-release, sustained boost. It mixes well with coconut in sweets to provide a very clear, wholesome treat. It is not unpleasant tasting, and has been compared to Horlicks and butterscotch because it has a kind of malty flavor. Not quite sweet, but not bitter either, it combines equally well in sweet and savory dishes. Maca powder starts to react once it is mixed with water, so if you are putting maca in your recipes be sure to eat them within a few days, or they get a strange, sickly aftertaste.

Like aloe vera and suma, maca is an adaptogen. This is a term coined by scientists in the 1930s to describe a plant that has a non-specific reaction in the body, and no harmful side effects. Adaptogens provide the body with "adaptation energy" and enable it to resist whatever stresses it is under and pressures it is suffering from. Thus adaptogens assist the body in maintaining homeostasis, a state of inner balance and core strength. This is why when you read about these plants, it sounds like they are good for everything. Aloe vera is reputed to help with immune system disorders like lupus and HIV, gut imbalances like colitis, Crohn's disease and IBS, skin conditions eczema and psoriasis, respiratory problems, joint inflammations, as well as being anti-aging and immune-boosting. Directly, it is not treating any of these ailments. But indirectly, it goes to where the body needs it, it gives strength to the body and promotes self-healing. That is why adaptogens are so powerful: they are getting to the very root cause of the symptoms, not trying to treat the outward signs of disease, but enabling the body to rebalance and dissolve the patterns that are creating the disease. They are dealing with cause rather than effect. Once health challenges are dealt with in this way, they are much less likely to reoccur than when only the outward manifestations of bad health are addressed and the inner roots left untouched.

Nutritionally, maca is a brilliant source of the B vitamin group including the elusive B12. The B vitamins are depleted in the body by stress; taking a food high in B vitamins like maca, pollen or gojis helps the body recover more quickly from stress and keep moving forward. The twenty-first-century lifestyle is a very stressful one due to environmental pollution and the fast-paced lives we lead; these superfoods are so valuable in giving us that energy to keep on keeping on, meet the demands placed on us, and rise to the challenges life presents us with. Maca is a good source of bioavailable protein, containing 11% amino

acids, and 18 out of the 22 amino acids needed to build protein in the body. It contains 31 different minerals and trace minerals, including significant amounts of calcium, magnesium, potassium, copper, zinc, iron, phosphorous, selenium and manganese, all of which are in a readily accessible form to the body. These minerals can help protect against osteoporosis, especially in menopausal women. The cruciferous family of vegetables is known for the glucosinates it contains, that have been demonstrated to have anti-cancer properties and inhibit tumor growth. The plant sterols in maca, like those in aloe vera, can be used as a natural and healthy alternative to steroid drugs, boosting performance for athletes, and helping the body fight challenges such as eczema. It helps with chronic fatigue not only because it provides healthy balanced energy levels, but also because it assists the adrenal glands and raises cortisol levels. Maca also provides many fatty acids, including lauric acid and linoleic acid (also known as omega-3, the EFA in which many of us are deficient).

As maca is a hormone balancer, it is beneficial for women at any time of their lives: if you have been on the pill, if you have irregular periods, if you suffer with premenstrual tension, if you have exceptionally light or heavy periods, if you are pregnant or breastfeeding, if you are entering adolescence, if you are premenopausal, in the menopause or postmenopausal. There are very few women that don't fit into one of those categories! Because it is rich in bioavailable calcium, it is particularly beneficial for breastfeeding mothers because it will balance your hormones, provide you with your extra calcium intake, and help you deal with all those sleepless nights. As a hormone balancer, it is also known as Nature's Viagra. It improves libido in both men and women, and also improves fertility. Maca and cacao together are an indisputable aphrodisiac. Maca does not itself contain hormones, so there is no danger of overdoing it. Rather, it supports the body's endocrine system which produces the hormones. The hypothalamus is the master gland that stimulates and balances the other glands in the body, and is also considered to be the brain's sex center; the beneficial effects maca has on the hypothalamus gland are central to its adaptogenic properties and aphrodisiacal effects. Maca also contains alkaloids which have been shown to increase fertility in humans—in a study done in 2000, the sexual activity of rats fed maca increased by 400%!

Children love maca. It is not unpalatable, and easily mixes into their cereal, porridge, or yogurt. It boosts their protein and calcium levels, building strength in the bones and teeth. As a hormone regulator, it can help prevent toddler tantrums, which are often just a result of hormonal surges overwhelming little bodies. It makes them strong, sure and confident in their bodies. When my children first had maca, they literally started climbing the walls! Reuben discovered how to straddle the door frame and climb it to reach the ceiling, and would show off his newfound skills to any and all visitors to our house. I'm also finding it very useful as they enter their teenage years, as a powerful way to lift them up out some of that teenage angst and returning them to good spirits.

Maca is so much more than the sum of its nutritive value. It is the actual energy of the plant that we are ingesting that has such a powerful effect on us holistically. Sure, it is a great source of protein, minerals, and plant sterols. But it is that adaptogenic effect, that "survival against all odds" element that it contains in its cells, that is so beneficial to us in the West at this time in history, when we are battling against so much within our culture, and trying to adapt to the new millennium unfolding before us. That's what makes maca magic!

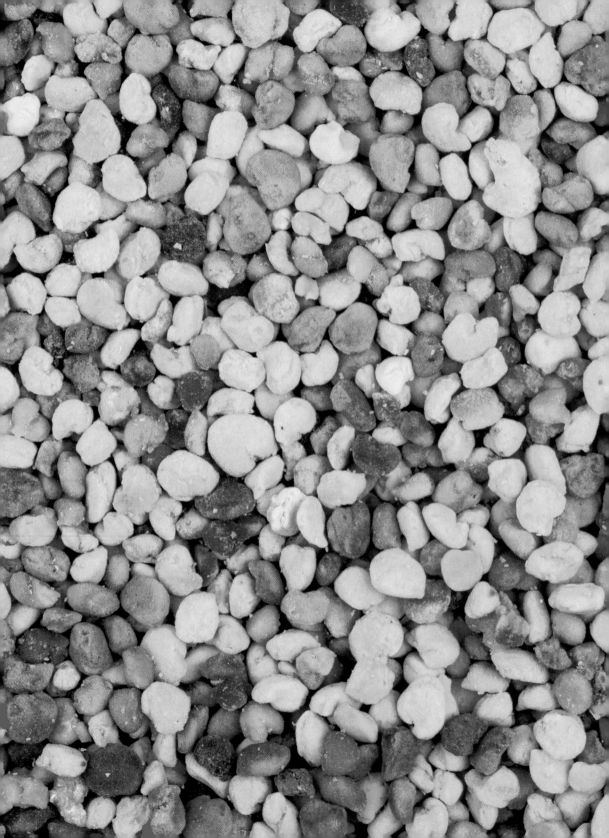

Pollen

Like algae, bee pollen is a perfect food, in that it contains every single known nutrient that the body needs. Theoretically, if you were stranded on a desert island, you could live on bee pollen and water alone. Pollen is also like algae in that it is a primordial food, one of the oldest foods on this planet, and so it must be made of something pretty amazing to have made it this far. Probably more has been written about pollen than any other food in this book; its incredible healing and rejuvenative properties are well researched and documented. Like all the superfoods, it is the synergistic effect of so many important nutrients that makes pollen so powerful, but it also contains substances as yet unidentified by science that add to its unique magic. Bee pollen is actually a bit of a misnomer because pollen does not come from bees, it comes from flowers, and is collected by the bees and brought back to the hives. Strictly speaking, pollen is not a vegan food, but I personally feel it is unlikely that Mother Nature would have designed the perfect food for humans and not meant us to eat it.

Pollen is a great superfood because it tastes so nice, sweet and rich like honey. Children love it, it is a wonderful food to add to their diets and increase their nutritional intake. It is easy to sprinkle on cereal for breakfast or add to trail mixes and desserts. Pollen has a very "buzzy" energy; it is sometimes called natural speed. I remember the first time I took it; it was about 10 p.m. at night, I had just put two children to bed, I was home on my own, and didn't know how I was going to face the rest of the evening's chores, tidying the kitchen and sorting out the washing. I took two pollen tablets to get me through those last few hours, and ended up with enough energy afterwards to dance around the living room! Pollen is a great food if you are always on the go, flitting from one activity to the next like a bee flying from flower to flower. If you are eating a meal that is a quick stopgap, with no time to rest or think, then adding pollen to it gives you that boost to rush off, full of enthusiasm and energy, rather than dragging yourself on feeling tired and reluctant.

The quality of bee pollen can be quite variable, and depends a lot on where it is gathered. Ideally, the environment in which the flowers and bees are living should be as pristine as possible, which is why desert pollen is very good. At one of the world's largest pollen producers, workers drive around the land in electric cars so as to minimize pollution. As a fresh food, pollen goes rancid easily. If it is kept in packaging that exposes it to light for long periods of time the quality can deteriorate. It also doesn't like being exposed to heat so it is best kept refrigerated. *You can tell if it is past its best by putting pollen granules in a glass of water—if it floats, it's rancid.* The majority of pollen that is sold in the West is dried—if you can find fresh pollen it's really in a class of its own. Look out for the French Percie du Sert pollen that is sold frozen to preserve it. Pollen also goes off quickly when it is ground up, so if you are adding it to recipes, better to use it in its whole form, unless you are planning on eating it straightaway. Most commercially available pollen is polyfloral, i.e. it comes from more than one variety of flower. Monofloral pollen is made when the bees collect pollen from one type of flower only, linden or hawthorn for example. Monofloral pollens have quite distinct tastes, and act on specific physical and energetic areas according to the flowers that they are from; for example, linden pollen is calming for the nerves, hawthorn nourishes the heart. The most beneficial pollen is that which is sourced locally to you, because then it is helping your body to tune into its immediate environment.

Pollen is produced by flowers and collected by bees that bind it with enzymes and carry it back to the hive in their pollen sacs. Beekeepers place fine brushes at the entrance to the hive that brush the bees' legs as they enter releasing the pollen from the sac, to later be collected by the beekeepers. Bees seek out the most nutritious pollen, so flowers compete for bees' attention as a means of ensuring their survival. In order to achieve reproductive success, flowers try to produce the most nutrient-dense pollen possible which ensures that pollen is always of the highest possible quality. Interestingly, when scientists have tried to replicate pollen in laboratories, by taking all pollen's known constituents and mixing them together, they have been unable. Bees in the hive live on pollen, but bees fed on this replicated pollen die. This proves that pollen contains some unidentifiable substances that must contribute to its special potency.

Pollen can help with allergies and hay fever. When taken at least six weeks before the beginning of hay fever season, symptoms are very much reduced. This works in a similar way to homeopathy: minute doses of the substance the body is allergic to builds up resistance so that when the body is exposed to larger doses, an immune response has been cultivated and no symptoms occur. The airborne pollen that people have a problem with is known as anemophile pollen grains; the kind that is collected by the bees is the entomophile pollen grains. Pollen has been shown in studies to have the same immune-strengthening results with other allergic reactions such as asthma and sinusitis. Because it is rich in enzymes, people often find pollen gives them digestive discomfort when they first take it because it is so stimulating to the gut. If this is the case, it is best to take it alone rather than with other foods, and consider a course of enemas or colonics because it is likely that old matter in the gut is being stirred up. Many people also find they are allergic to pollen. Out of all the foods in this book, pollen is the one people are most likely to have a problem with; people commonly report itchy skin or tingly lips. This is due in part to the fact that we all have weakened immune systems due to antibiotic use, pollution in the environment, poor diets and not enough exposure to nature. If this is the case, you can either fast to cleanse the system before trying pollen again, or just build up slowly. If you keep taking minute amounts of pollen daily, your resistance will build up and you can gradu-ally increase the dose until your immune system functioning is restored and the pollen doesn't have the same detoxify-ing effect.

Bee pollen's use goes way back into history. It is recommended in the Bible, as well as by Pliny, Pythagoras, and Hippocrates. It is also mentioned in ancient Chinese and Egyptian texts. In Russia, where pollen has been much researched, inhabitants of the villages near the Caucasus Mountains are renowned for their longevity, with many centenarians living amongst them. In the 1970s, some American scientists investigated into the cause of their extraordinary longevity, and found that there were many bee-keepers among them, and the common factor was the "scrap honey" they all ate, the residue from the bottom of the hive, rich in pollen, propolis and other beneficial substances. Like royal jelly, another popular therapeutic bee product, pollen is well regarded for its anti-aging properties, as it stimulates cell renewal and so rejuvenates the skin.

Pollen contains at least 96 nutritional elements. It contains all 22 amino acids, consisting of 40% protein, weight for weight more than any animal product. Bee pollen is a great dietary source of B vitamins. Whenever we get stressed because we are doing too much, our B vitamin levels get depleted, so taking pollen is an excellent antidote to stress. If we have had a stressful incident in our day, for instance getting stuck in a traffic jam and then not having enough time to get ready for an important meeting, or having an argument with someone and then having to take the children out somewhere, taking some pollen gives us the energy to carry on without feeling depleted. It is one of the best dietary sources of vitamin B6, and a reputed source of the hard-to-find B12. It is a good source of vitamin C, the best dietary source of rutin, a glucoside that strengthens the capillary system, and one of the richest sources of carotenoids and bioflavonoids. Pollen is a great source of minerals, especially zinc. It has significant amounts of potassium, calcium, phosphorous, magnesium, silicon, manganese, sulphur, selenium and iron.

Here are some more of the benefits of pollen:

- As far back as 1948, research was published that showed that taking bee pollen acts as a preventative against cancer, and can reduce tumors. It has also been demonstrated to protect against radiation and help with the side effects of chemotherapy.

- Pollen is good for fertility; it is literally the sperm of the flower, the male seed produced in large quantities to ensure some of it succeeds in carrying on the species. It stimulates the ovaries and improves the libido. Due in addition to its high zinc content, it is particularly good for prostrate problems.

- It is favored by athletes for its abilities to increase stamina and endurance, and was used by Muhammad Ali to "float like a butterfly, sting like a bee." There are many, many reports from sportspeople and sports trainers who have used bee pollen to improve their performance.

- It is rich in lecithin, which helps to metabolize fats in the body. Lecithin contains substantial amounts of phosphatidyl choline, which is beneficial for the brain, especially for children whose brains are still developing. For this reason also, it is a great food for pregnant women. Bee pollen has great synergy with flax oil, because the lecithin in the pollen helps ensure flax oil's abundant supply of EFAs are broken down and absorbed properly.

- It is a great source of the nucleic acids RNA and DNA, the building blocks of the body.

- Like coconut oil, it normalizes cholesterol levels in the blood and balances the metabolism, so helping with weight loss.

- Like algae, it is a superb source of phenylananine, which regulates the body's natural appetite.

- It rehabilitates the gut, strengthens the intestines, and has been used to treat Crohn's disease, colitis, and digestive ulcers.

- It is a natural antibiotic.

- It is popular for pets, for boosting their immune systems, improving the quality of their coats, increasing longevity and as an aid to fertility.

- It has been used to treat anemia, it boosts the circulation, aids cardiovascular health, regulates the blood sugar, and has been extremely successful at treating a huge variety of weaknesses and illnesses.

- Taking locally harvested fresh bee pollen is far superior to the dried stuff, if you can find it. Taking local pollen can help combat allergies from flowers and dust in the area from which it is harvested.

Pollen and cacao together is a brilliant source of positive energy. When you eat pollen and cacao, you feel like you can do anything! As pollen has a natural sweetness, it complements the bitterness of the cacao well. We often make trail mix just by mixing up some pollen granules and nibs up with a few other snack foods like goji berries, coconut chips, or yacon root.

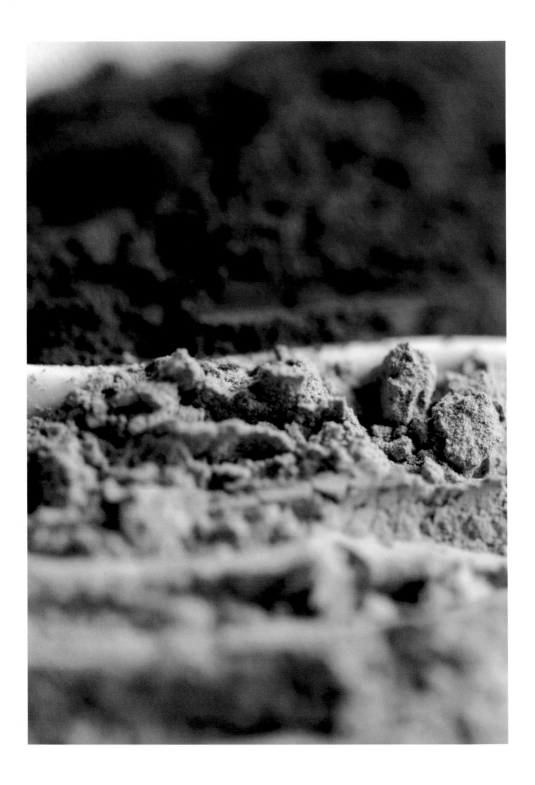

Raw Magic

The Algaes

"Spirulina can help restore our lives. It's the next best thing to eating sunlight! Eat algae and bring light into your own cells. Consume less and live lighter on the Earth. Magnified by millions of people, life begins to change. This is a magnificent legacy for our next generations."
—ROBERT HENRIKSON, FOUNDER OF THE WORLD'S LARGEST SPIRULINA FARM

There are three types of nutritionally dense algae commonly consumed in the UK: spirulina, Klamath Lake blue-green algae, and chlorella. My personal preference is for Klamath Lake algae because it is a wild food, and I believe it is important to consume as many wild foods as we can on a daily basis. Wild foods provide us with a direct connection to the earth, their natural state hasn't been tampered with, they are more whole, and so have a stronger vitality. Spirulina and chlorella are both farmed algaes. However spirulina is considerably cheaper, and more suitable for eating in large amounts, so if you're going for bulk, then spirulina would be a better choice. I would rarely eat more than one teaspoon of Klamath Lake algae at a time, whereas I often eat several tablespoons of spirulina in a guacamole or a smoothie. Chlorella is not so readily available as spirulina and Klamath

Lake algae, and is most often found in tablet form.

The algaes are one of the most nutrient dense foods known to man, and the highest vegetable source of vitamin B12. Algae are a purely natural plant food, going through minimal processing to reach us in edible form. Algae were the initial life form on earth, and blue-green algae dates back over four billion years. There is evidence to show that algae were one of man's first foods: races such as the Aztecs and Incas harvested and ate raw algae. Tribes in Africa still depend on algae for their sustenance, and algae have been used in Chinese medicine throughout the centuries. When we eat algae, we are connecting with a profound and ancient energy. Richard France, a macrobiotic counselor, states, "It is not inconceivable that on subtle vibrational levels, unique genetic memories and messages of harmony and peace are stored in algae, which have grown undisturbed for years in a pristine environment. This information may be passed to us at a cellular level, encouraging harmony among our own cellular family."

Not only do algae contain a high density of vitamins and minerals, as well as many other health-giving properties, algae have an assimilation rate of over 90%, which means that all these nutrients are readily absorbed and used by the body. Many nutrients from laboratory-formulated supplements are wasted as they are in a form that cannot be utilized by the body. Many nutrients work with each other. For example, the body needs adequate levels of vitamin C to absorb iron, so when iron supplements are taken on their own, they are ineffective if the correct levels of vitamin C are not present in the diet. However, in blue-green algae, we find the ideal balance of nutrients for our needs. If you were going to design the perfect food for humans, with every single nutrient present in optimum ratios, it would have a remarkably similar nutritional profile to these algaes.

Algae contain:

- All the essential trace minerals: boron, calcium, chromium, cobalt, copper, iron, magnesium, manganese, phosphorous, potassium, sodium, zinc and vanadium, in perfect balance for optimum health.

- Vitamins thiamine (B1), riboflavin (B2), pyrodoxine (B6), niacin (B3), vitamin B12, vitamin C, choline, pantothenic acid (B5), biotin, folic acid, and vitamin E, also in exactly the right balance for maximum bioavailability. Although algae manufacturers will testify that the B12 in their products is assimilable by the body, recent research by Gabriel Cousens has indicated that the B12 in spirulina, Klamath Lake algae and nori are analogues and do not meet our nutritional requirements.

- All eight amino acids, and in a form more easily digested by the body than those found in meat and vegetable protein (85% assimilable, whereas beef is only 20% assimilable).

- Thousands of live active enzymes. Enzymes are a little-mentioned component of health, yet vital to every process of the body. They are completely destroyed by temperatures of over 118°C: consequently, all cooked food is devoid of enzymes, and many of us may be lacking in sufficient amounts to ensure vitality, especially in winter months when our intake of fruit and salads tends to be lower. A daily dose of blue-green algae can be invaluable in providing us with some of this precious resource.

- The highest source of chlorophyll in the plant kingdom, as well as other health-giving pigments. Chlorophyll is an amazing healer, and helps to correct overacidity in the body. I provide more information on chlorophyll in the chapter on wheatgrass. The presence of chlorophyll is one of the elements that make algae such a great detoxification food. Taking algae has been shown to assist in removing heavy metals from the body. In 1993, studies showed it had beneficial effects on children from Chernobyl suffering from radiation sickness.

- RNA/DNA, nucleic acids essential in the reparation of cells and growth of body tissue.

- Essential fatty acids. These fats are vital to good health, but as they are only found in fish, and seeds such as flax and hemp, they are often lacking in a vegan diet.

- One of the highest known natural sources of beta-carotene, a rich source of vitamin A.

They can be used on a daily basis, simply to sustain good health, but they have also been used to treat conditions such as IBS, Alzheimer's disease, anemia, hypoglycemia, liver fatigue, depression, and candida. They have been proven to aid concentration and memory, strengthen the immune system, and counteract over-acidity in the body. They enhance cardiovascular health and reduce cholesterol levels, and have been used in the treatment of serious illnesses such as cancer and AIDS. International research has been going on into spirulina for decades, and there is much evidence to support these health claims. Unlike many health foods, where there is no funding made available for research, manufacturers who see the huge economic potential of chlorella and spirulina as a retail product have commissioned many in-depth, scientific papers.

Spirulina is a farmed algae, produced mainly in Hawaii and China. It grows at very fast rates, and provides more nutrition per acre than any other crop on the planet. It can even be grown in the irrigation beds in rice fields. As such, it is one of the most ecologically responsible and sustainable foods available. Under a microscope, it looks like green spiraling threads, hence the name. It is a very hardy plant, and can adapt and grow in many different environments, thus it provides us with that ability to adapt and thrive in adverse conditions. Spirulina contains over 60% protein; per acre, that means you can grow 20 times more protein than soya beans, and 200 times more than beef!

Chlorella is so named because of its exceptionally high chlorophyll content. It is a single-celled algae which is cultivated mainly in Asia. In Japan, it is eaten by seven million people daily, and is more popular than vitamin C supplements! What singles out chlorella from the other algae is the Chlorella Growth Factor, or CGF. The entire reproductive cycle of chlorella can take place in 24 hours given the right conditions. What the CGF factor exactly is remains a bit of a mystery. But it means it is effective at cell restoration, tissue repair, and is very beneficial for growing children.

Klamath Lake blue-green algae are currently one of the few wild, uncultivated strains of algae growing in the world. It is harvested from the Upper Klamath Lake in Oregon, U.S.A. The Klamath Lake basin acts as a "nutrient trap" for the surrounding 4,000 square miles of secluded wilderness in the Cascade Mountains. Seventeen rivers and streams feed the lake with a rich supply of minerals, volcanic silt and many other nutrients. So pure are their waters that the locals refer to them as "The Rivers of Light." To get the maximum benefits from algae it is vital that it does not reach extreme temperatures during processing; heating or freezing will destroy it. Look for algae that have been flash-dried, as this leaves the cells of the algae intact and retains its bioactivity.

Klamath Lake algae are also an invaluable addition to a child's diet. As any parent knows, it can be a challenge trying to strike a balance between a child's fussy habits and meeting their nutritional needs. Algae are great for children because you need such small amounts: just ¼ teaspoon a day can be smuggled into their favorite foods, and acts like a kind of safety net in meeting their nutritional needs, ensuring their health and your peace of mind. Algae are also great to feed your pets. It is reported to improve their coats and hair, and increase longevity. My cats go crazy for chlorella tablets!

Klamath Lake algae come in many different forms: liquid, powdered, tablets or capsules. E3-Live is a specially freeze-dried algae which comes in liquid form to preserve its nutritional properties. My favorite way of taking it is in its potentiated form, either as Crystal Manna, or E3 AFA. Crystal Manna is one of the most out-of-this-world foods I have ever come across—green and sparkly, it looks just like fairy dust. If you think of Masaru Emoto's book *The Hidden Messages in Water*, and imagine your cells to be snowflakes, every one is a crystal like that. Our bodies are mostly water, after all, and everything we put in our bodies is going to affect our snowflakes. If we eat food that has been mass-produced, with all the life taken out of it, that is going to damage our snowflakes and make them into chaotic and distorted patterns. But when we eat superfoods, their vital energy is so strong they help our snowflakes become beautiful. Crystal Manna is such a beautiful food, when I eat it I feel like my snowflakes are crystallizing into amazing patterns—literally, I feel sparkly!

Blue Manna, or E3 AFA Mend, is another favorite way to consume algae. Blue Manna is the blue pigment extracted from Klamath Lake algae. This extract is very rich in PEA and phycocyanin. As we discussed in the chapter on cacao, PEA is known as "the molecule of joy." It is naturally produced in the brain when we are in states of bliss, totally involved in an activity that we love. It makes us completely present, lost in the moment, oblivious of outside distractions. PEA is a great brain food. It sharpens the mind, and creates clear, focused intelligence. Phycocyanin is a natural anti-inflammatory, and very beneficial for the joints. Taking Blue Manna every day helps us keep sharp and on the button. Because of the pathways it creates in the brain, it leads us to make choices that are following our bliss, empowering us creatively, rather than ignoring the gifts and talents of our heart, or feeling scared of taking decisions that inspire us. Of course, algae contains PEA and phycocyanin, so just taking algae will ensure you get these elements in your diet, but Blue Manna enables you to receive them in a more concentrated form.

Wheatgrass and Barleygrass

"Wheatgrass juice is the nectar of rejuvenation, the plasma of youth, the blood of all life. The elements that are missing in your body's cells—especially enzymes, vitamins, hormones, and nucleic acids—can be obtained through this daily green sunlight transfusion."
—VIKTORAS KULVINSKAS, AUTHOR SURVIVAL IN THE 21ST CENTURY

Wheatgrass and barleygrass are virtually identical. They are among the most alkaline foods available. As such, they are very calming, nurturing and purifying.

They are most commonly consumed freshly juiced, or in powdered form. Growing your own wheatgrass and juicing it yourself is one of the most powerful cleansing techniques known in the alternative health field. Anne Wigmore first popularized the use of wheatgrass for therapeutic purposes back in the 1930s. She tried a variety of different grasses, and found wheatgrass to be the most beneficial. Along with Viktoras Kulvinskas, she founded the Hippocrates Health Institute in Boston. Now run by Brian and Maria Clements in Florida, Hippocrates is world-renowned for healing people with apparently terminal illnesses. They have countless testimonials from patients who have been given no hope by their doctors, people suffering from heart disease, cancer and diabetes. Using a living foods program with large doses of wheatgrass as a central plank of the regimen, they have nurtured thousands back to optimum health.

The use of barley, for food and nutritional purposes, dates back to ancient times. Roman gladiators ate barley for strength and stamina. In the West, it was first known for the barley grain it produces. Barley grass contains 18 amino eight contains a variety of vitamins and minerals, including beta-carotene, folic acid, vitamins C, E and five B vitamins (including B12), calcium, iron, magnesium, and phosphorus. Barley grass is said to have 30 times as much vitamin B1 and eleven times the amount of calcium as cow's milk; three times as much vitamin C, six times as much carotene and nearly five times as much iron as spinach; nearly seven times the vitamin C of oranges and four times the vitamin B1 of whole wheat flour.

Wheatgrass contains 20% protein, which includes a balanced blend of 20 amino acids, and nearly double the amount of beta-carotene found in carrots. It is one of the best sources of chlorophyll available. It contains over 90 trace minerals. Drinking 1 oz wheatgrass juice is the nutritional equivalent of eating 1 kg fresh vegetables! As such, it's the ultimate convenience food, a surefire way to get your daily requirements in. Because it is in juice form, it is instantly absorbable by the cells, ensuring maximum assimilation. People sometimes worry that if they have an intolerance to wheat, they will not be able to consume wheatgrass. Most people who avoid wheat do so because of the high gluten content of the grain once it has been cooked. In raw wheat grain, the starches turn to sugars when they sprout, so there is no gluten content. Unless you are celiac, a condition that means you should avoid all wheat products entirely, wheatgrass is a safe and beneficial health choice.

As well as their excellent nutritional profiles, the grasses carry first-class enzymes into the cells when they are consumed freshly harvested. They have been shown to neutralize and digest the toxins in our cells. Consequently, they have antiseptic, antibacterial and deodorizing properties. They contain an enzyme that increases resistance to radiation, and is used on people suffering from radiation sickness. The grasses can also be used externally due to their high antioxidant capabilities. They are great for the skin and hair, and are sometimes used as poultices. They can relieve the irritation of eczema, psiorasis, sunburn, and are used for all types of wound healing—bites, stings, cuts, sores, and boils. Chewing wheatgrass or applying it to the infected area can help with toothache and freshens the breath. You can even put it in the bath!

Wheatgrass is so simple and easy to grow. All you need is organic wheat grain, organic compost and a seed tray with a lid. Soak half a cup (60 g/2 oz) of wheat grain overnight, and then in the morning, drain and leave to sprout for around 12 hours. When it's ready, spread a layer of compost on the seed tray, and spread the seed evenly over the top. Water, and cover with the lid. Leave it in a warm, light place for four days, by which time you will have green shoots starting to show. After four days, remove the lid and water daily for another three days, by which time you should have a luscious green crop. If you have a high-power juicer, you can push the grass straight through; one tray should make about 8 oz grass. If you have a high-power blender, put a handful in the blender jug with a glass of water and blend for a couple of minutes. Strain and serve. If you don't have either of these pieces of equipment, you can just chew the grass and spit out the fiber, which is indigestible. By harvesting the grass before it forms a seed, you are consuming it when it's at its peak, its nutritional level at its highest. It is recommended to start with just a 1 oz shot of wheatgrass juice every day, and work your way up to 2 oz. Most people consider 2 oz enough!

A fantastic way to detox is to drink a shot of wheatgrass or barleygrass juice for breakfast every morning. It makes most people feel sick—this is the liver cleansing and releasing bile. If you try wheatgrass and it doesn't make you ill, don't big yourself up too much! It's more likely that the toxins are deeply buried and you're not absorbing the grass properly. Keep drinking it every morning, and chances are, within a few days, you'll be wanting to retch! The best way to think of wheatgrass is like medicine—it's not going to taste nice, but you know it's going to make you feel good. It took years of drinking it at least three times a week before it stopped making me nauseous. But I still looked forward to it because I knew once I'd got it down me, I'd feel calmer, clearer and cleaner.

The powders aren't as effective, and are much more costly, but are still a brilliant way to alkalize your diet. Barleygrass powder has quite a pleasant, sweet-edged taste, which makes it more palatable to add to recipes. If you read the ingredients lists on the labels, you'll see that many of the superfood blends on the market are mainly barleygrass or wheatgrass powder, or sometimes spirulina. They are usually expensive because you are paying for the development of the blend, and all the packaging and marketing. Buying pure barleygrass or wheatgrass powder is a much more economical way of getting these green superfoods in you. You can also obtain frozen juices. Freezing destroys a little of the enzymatic content and nutritional properties, so it's not as beneficial as fresh juice, but still better than none at all. One way to take the juice is to make a whole tray of it, then put it into ice cube trays in the freezer. You can add these cubes to drinks, so you just get a flavor of grass in your drink, or defrost a couple and drink them neat.

People often raise the contradiction between recommending locally grown foods and seasonal eating, and promoting superfoods, as I do. My feeling is that ideally, we would all be eating foods picked wild from the surrounding area. But the modern-day diet is so far from that point, we need some assistance getting back to the ideal. Due to unsustainable farming techniques, and environmental pollution, our food lacks the potency and mineral qualities that it once had. The superfoods act as a bridge; they are intense foods that help restore our nutritional balance and give us the brain fuel to make the right choices to get back to an ideal lifestyle. But wheatgrass and barleygrass are the ultimate superfoods because they fulfill both criteria. When you grow your own grass, it costs pennies, and uses minimal resources. You can put your loving energy into the grass as you grow it, so you know that it's never been maltreated. When you juice it fresh, it's 100% alive, all the enzymatic activity is intact, and you know it's not been depleted by traveling halfway across the world.

The magic in the grasses lies in the fact that chlorophyll is the most similar substance to human blood known. It's identical but for the fact that the iron molecule present in haemoglobin is replaced by magnesium in chlorophyll. Magnesium is a mineral that most of us lack in our diets. So when you drink wheatgrass juice, which is 70% chlorophyll, you are literally drinking green blood, plant blood. You are oxygenating your blood, cleansing out all the rubbish and restoring your cells to their natural state of perfection. Chlorophyll is the basis of all plant life, it is the first product of light, so when you drink fresh juice you are effectively drinking liquid light. When you set yourself up with such a strong cleanser first thing in the morning, that has a powerful knock-on effect on the rest of your food choices for the day. Wheatgrass balances the blood sugar, so you're less prone to mood swings. Fewer emotional ups and downs mean you're less likely to reach for the junk food when you have a dip. A balanced blood sugar also knocks sugar cravings on the head. Before I started drinking wheatgrass daily, I had a passion for dates. Fresh dates were one of my favorite treats, a comfort food when I was feeling knocked-out. Dates are a good source of minerals, but extremely destabilizing to blood sugar levels. As I started consuming fresh grass daily, I noticed dates started to taste over-sweet to me. Before long, I lost my craving for them completely. If you are having problems with candida, wheatgrass is one of the best ways to kill sugar cravings and help you stick with a low-glycemic diet. These effects also help with weight management. Once you've drunk your wheatgrass, eating is usually the last thing you feel like doing while your body processes and cleanses. And once it's done its work and rebalanced your blood, you're going to feel revitalized, and far less likely to reach for the snacks. Put a clean liver, a balanced blood sugar and an even emotional keel all together, and you've got guaranteed weight-loss. So like all the superfoods, the power of the grasses can't be measured just in their nutritive value. They have a deeper effect on our energy and consciousness that will ripple out to all areas of our daily lives.

Purple Corn Extract, Suma and Camu Camu and More...

These very special foods were largely unheard of in the West until recently. Like the monatomic trace elements, they are virtually a cross between vibrational essences and foods. You need to take them in almost homeopathic doses to feel the effects: it is as much about getting the vibration of the plant into your body as experiencing the nutritional benefits. In fact, these foods are so potent that large doses can be detrimental, having such an extreme effect on the body. The first time we had purple corn extract, we shared one teaspoon between six of us, and were amazed at the noticeable difference we felt.

Purple corn extract comes from the Amazon. It is a rare strain of normal maize, and different from the blue corn found in some breads and tortilla chips. In Mayan cultures it is a revered and sacred plant central to their mythology. An ancient Mayan prophecy says that when purple corn extract comes to the West, it will be the shift between the ages, the time of remembrance. Purple corn extract is said to activate the ancient cellular memory, and reconnect us with the wisdom of our DNA. Purple is the color of the pituitary gland, the third eye, the color of psychoactive awareness,

seeing beyond the veil into the unseen world. Many people believe that to eat holistically is to eat a rainbow diet that includes all colors of the spectrum in our diet. The colors of the lower chakras, red, orange, yellow, and green are easy, but blues, purples and pinks are often lacking. Just getting that purple ray into our diet can fill a part of us we weren't even aware we were lacking. Purple corn extract is mainly grown in Peru. It is one of the best dietary sources of anthocyanins, the potent antioxidant found in blueberries. This antioxidant reduces cholesterol and is a natural anti-inflammatory. It has a fruity flavor, and makes a wonderful addition to any dish, sweet or savory, that you want to add a purple tinge to. In Peru they make a drink with it called *chicha morada*. Please note that many raw food companies sell purple corn extract flour. The flour is simply the whole kernel ground down, and is not anywhere near as tasty or beneficial. You want to seek out the extract, which is a concentrated form of anthocyanins, and is a deep dark purple color.

Camu camu came along to steal the crown from the goji berry as contender for the fruit with the most vitamin C on the planet, containing a whopping 2 g of vitamin C in every 100 g of fruit. This may not sound like a lot compared to the amount that is in a high potency vitamin C supplement, but because the vitamin C in camu camu is concentrated it means it works in synergy for maximum benefit. It is a berry that grows on shrubs in the Amazon rainforest, and looks similar to grapes. It is a powerhouse of phytochemicals, including amino acids, minerals like calcium, potassium, and iron, the B group of vitamins, and beta-carotene. It can be used as an antidepressant, to treat ADD, and herpes. The high amounts of vitamin C it contains make it antiviral, and help boost the immune system. Although clinical studies have been done, there is very little scientific research available on camu, and doubtless this plant contains many exciting properties we have yet to discover. We find camu camu energizing, cleansing and refreshing. It tastes a little like lemon sherbet, and is a great way to balance out the sweetness of cakes and puddings.

Suma is a vine with an intricate root system that grows in the Amazon rainforest. It is one of the most powerful foods in this book, and also one of the most difficult to describe. In Brazil, it is known as *Para Toda*, which means "for all things." Like aloe vera and maca, suma is an adaptogen, that is, it assists the body in restoring homeostasis and creates balance and harmony without any detrimental side effects. Adaptogens have a normalizing effect on the body, and can be taken daily for long periods of time without overstimulating the system. In our experience, suma is such a potent adaptogen, it is a medicine for the soul. It shakes us right back into our central core, and reminds us of ways in our lives that we are out of sync with ourselves. It shines a light on dark corners of our personalities that are neglected and hidden. Suma contains a strong plant spirit, and is practically shamanic in its effects. A quarter of a teaspoon is all that is needed to get the energy of the plant into you. Larger doses are not usually advised! Its effect is so individualized, it is impossible to say what it will do for you. I have had reports of people taking it and having so much energy they have had to go for a run, or do some martial arts; other people take it and are knocked to the floor, feeling so dreamy and relaxed they can barely move. If you are the sort of person who is always busy and doesn't slow down enough, then suma is likely to chill you out; if you are too chilled out already and need a bit of get up and go, suma will do that for you instead. It reminds you that that side of yourself exists, and that is a wonderful place to be too.

Like cacao, suma enhances the effects of other foods, which is why we like to add it to our chocolate and smoothies. As an adaptogen, suma works beneficially on the hormones, is great for PMS, the menopause, and acts on the libido. It contains most of the amino acids, minerals and trace minerals, including important amounts of germanium, and vitamins including the B group and vitamin E. It is thought that the high levels of germanium is one of the factors that make suma so potent: germanium oxygenates the body at the cellular level, and stimulates the immune system. Suma contains high levels of saponins, which have been used in the prevention of cancer, and to regulate blood pressure. Known as Brazilian ginseng, it was traditionally used for strength and endurance.

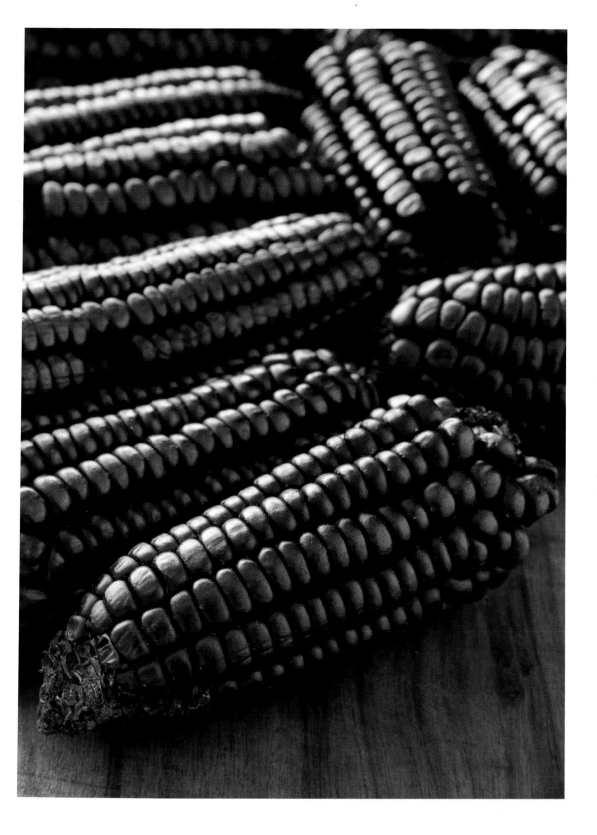

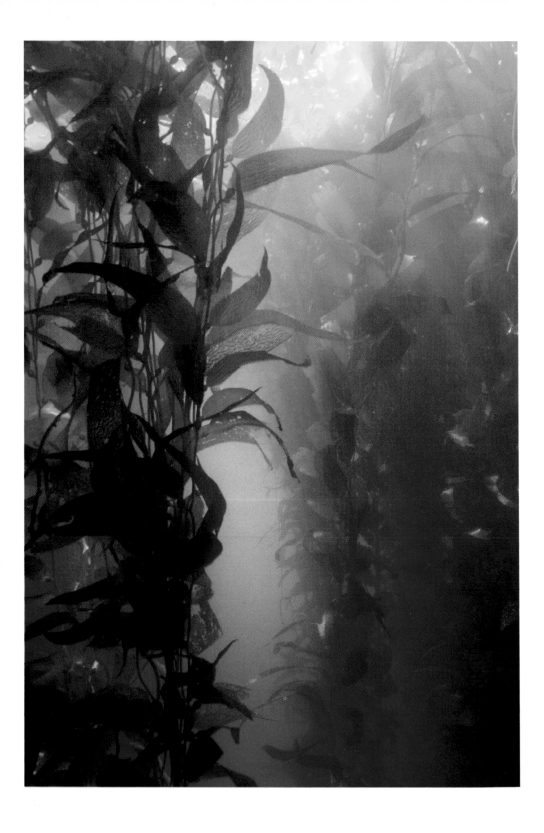

Sea Vegetables

"It may seem strange to be singing the praises of seaweed as a valuable source of minerals, then saying how it can be used to remove metals from the body. This is the paradox of a natural system, working both ways at the same time, removing imbalances, restoring things to the way they should be. Something that no modern wonder drug has ever managed to achieve."
—SONIA SUREY-GENT, MARINE BIOLOGIST

"I once heard a story about a certain village somewhere in Canada's Bay of Fundy area where everyone ate dulse. After a hundred years or so they had to shoot an old fellow just to start a graveyard. The same village went from a population of just over two people to over fifteen hundred in the shortest span of years that anyone ever witnessed. The first old fellow to die there was 101 at his time of death. Some say he would still be alive today if he had not drowned on the way to the hospital to try and remove the bullets. Don't laugh. His poor grandmother mourned at the gravesite every day for years."
—www.rolandsdulse.com

Seaweeds are an essential part of my daily diet. They are calming, rebalancing, mineralising, satisfying, and delicious. The earth's surface area is covered in over 70% sea; if we want to connect with the earth holistically, it is important to eat seafoods on a regular basis. Think of how you feel at the beach: uplifted, relaxed, expansive, energized, nourished. So when we eat the foods of the sea, we are absorbing that energy into our bodies. I make sure the family has them at every meal. Seaweeds nourish us in ways most foods don't because they are a wild food:

wild foods have all their vital force intact, they come direct from the earth, so make us feel connected, and provide us with that free and untamed energy that is so lacking in our sanitized, fearful Western culture.

Traditionally an integral part of Asian diets, sea vegetables are increasing in popularity here in the West as people start to recognize their extraordinary health benefits and versatility. In Japan they have been eaten for many thousands of years. They are also popular in Ireland, Iceland, France, Spain, Australia, Canada, Hawaii; indeed, most countries which have large coastal regions. When purchasing sea vegetables, pick out ones from a good quality brand who have been careful to harvest the produce from clean waters, and then dry them out for you with the appropriate care and attention. You can pick up sea vegetables at bargain prices from Asian grocers, although the quality is variable, and they are often roasted or fried, which might bring out the flavors but destroys some of the nutritional content. Incidentally, when you buy crispy seaweed in a Chinese shop or restaurant, this isn't seaweed at all but a deep-fried cabbage! There are thousands of varieties of sea vegetables, and they are usually classified by color—brown, red, or green. They are not technically a plant or a vegetable, but belong to the algae family. Because they are dried and can be kept in the cupboard until you are ready to eat them, they are such an easy food to use. Organic seaweeds are those that are guaranteed to have been harvested from unpolluted waters.

Since the Fukushima disaster, many people have been concerned about consuming Japanese sea vegetables. It's more important than ever that we only buy from suppliers who can guarantee the purity and quality of their product. I would be very wary of picking up any sea vegetables from an Asian grocer, and check with the manufacturer that your sea vegetables have been tested for radiation, with satisfactory results. They should be tested in Japan, and then again when they get to America.

Sea vegetables are just about the most mineral-rich foods available, being a brilliant source of the B-group of vitamins and vitamin K, as well as a good protein source. Although they don't contain all the essential amino acids, they do contain them in a form that is easily assimilated by the body. Indeed, all the nutrients in seaweeds are in a colloidal, balanced form, so they are very bioavailable. As a wild food, sea vegetables are a source of that elusive vitamin B12, although there is some debate as to how absorbable the B12 is to the body. They contain all of the trace minerals that can be lacking from land-grown foods due to soil depletion, essential minerals that we are often missing in our daily diet like selenium and chromium. They are a very low-calorific, high-fiber food that's great for maintaining weight. They are a fantastic source of iodine, an important mineral that is more or less absent from land vegetables. Iodine is essential for the healthy functioning of the thyroid gland, which controls our metabolism, and so also assists in regulating body weight. It is one of the best plant sources of calcium—half a cup of dulse or hijiki contains more calcium than a cup of milk, and is much more easily assimilated by the body. Sea vegetables have been demonstrated to provide the body with certain phyto-nutrients that inhibit tumor growth. They are a natural anti-inflammatory agent, due to the poly-saccharides they contain, and because of their high levels of magnesium and phy-to-nutrients, they can help relieve PMS. They are a perfect substitute for salt in the diet, containing healthy levels of sodium in the right balance for the human body. The naturally occurring glutamic acids in seaweed act as a flavor enhancer that complement the natural flavors of any dish.

Dulse The two most popular sea vege-tables among raw fooders are dulse and nori. Dulse is soft, purple seaweed. Unlike most sea vegetables, it needs no pre-soaking, just a quick rinse in fresh water to remove any stray shells and pebbles! It comes in two forms, the whole blade, or flakes, which are perfect as a salad gar-nish. Dulse is one of the few purple foods found in our diets. Purple is the psychoac-tive color, the color of the third eye, and we don't have enough of it in our diets. Like all the sea vegetables, it is rich in minerals; dulse is full of calcium, potas-sium, magnesium, and iron. Dulse is really good deep-fried and turned into crisps or you can make raw crisps in the dehydrator (there's a recipe in my book *Raw Living*). It adds a gorgeous richness when blended into tomato sauces. It is most commonly harvested from the Atlantic and Pacific oceans.

Nori comes either toasted or raw. The toasted sheets are dark green and are commonly found in Asian grocers. Nori rolls are like the raw-fooder's sandwich. You can put anything and everything in them, and roll them up for an instant and satisfying snack food. We also blend nori up into soups and sauces, where it acts as a thickening agent, or cut the sheets into small strips and add them to salads. You can buy nori flakes that go great as a garnish on just about anything. *Laver* is the name also given to the seaweed from which nori sheets are made. Such is its popularity that nori has been a cultivated food in Japan for over 300 years. Once it is harvested, it is washed and hung out on bamboo frames to dry in a process similar to papermaking. It is a reputed source of vitamin B12, and contains more protein than any of the other sea vegeta-bles, 40%.

Sea spaghetti is an incredible food, really similar to tagliatelle in appearance and texture, although obviously with a fishy flavor! Many people go mad for it when they first have it. It tastes as good as it is for you, containing some nutrients that the body finds hard to get elsewhere. There are some foods that when you eat them taste unique: avocados are one, or the Peruvian fruit lucuma is another. You just know instinctively that you are get-ting a great synergy of valuable nutrients that you can't find anywhere else. Sea spaghetti is a great source of the miner-als iron, calcium, magnesium, phospho-rous, and iodine, as well as all the essen-tial amino acids. It needs soaking for at least 30 minutes before eating.

Wakame is a leafy green seaweed that can be added to salads or used to thicken sauces. It is a particularly good source of magnesium. It needs soaking for ten min-utes before eating.

Arame has a mild, sweet taste. It has delicate, thin black fronds, similar to spaghetti. It needs soaking for ten minutes before eating. It is richest in iron and calcium.

Hijiki is a black sea vegetable, similar to arame in appearance but with thicker strands. It increases in volume to around four times its original size when soaked. It is one of the stronger tasting seaweeds, with an intense nutty flavor. It needs soaking for at least 20 minutes before eating. It does not come to us raw, but is steamed or boiled and then dried after harvesting. However, I believe sea vegetables are such an important part of our diet, it is better to eat them this way than not at all.

Kelp is a variety of kombu, usually sold in granular form. You can buy it as tablets, but we buy it loose and sprinkle it over our salads. It is the number one dietary source of iodine—8 g kelp contains 100% of the iodine RDA—so you only need a tiny bit every day. Just a quarter of a teaspoon on your food is not going to be noticed in taste, but will really boost your mineral intake. It's little things that this that make all the difference to maintaining a good health regimen and not sliding off the rails. Because of its high iodine content, kelp stimulates the thyroid, and is good for people who have an underactive thyroid condition. It is rich in iron, potassium, calcium and magnesium. The phytochemicals in kelp have been demonstrated to absorb radioactivity and heavy metals and remove them from the body. For this reason, they are a great detox food, and especially beneficial if you are having mercury fillings removed.

Kombu can be bought in whole strips and makes a great addition to cooking, although it is too tough to eat raw.

Bladderwrack is sold in the UK under the Seagreens brand. Wrack has a complete nutritional profile, that is, like wild blue-green algae and bee pollen, it contains every single identifiable nutrient that the body requires—and probably some we haven't identified too! Like kelp, it is excellent for removing heavy metals and toxins from the body, as it contains the polysaccharide fucoidan, and has been used to treat children with autism, who often have a mineral imbalance. Seagreens comes as granules, and is absolutely delicious sprinkled over salads or as a garnish for soups. If you can't track down Seagreens, you can substitute any kind of sea vegetable granules in the recipes; Maine Coast does a great range in the USA.

Irish moss is a sea vegetable that I wasn't so familiar with when I wrote the recipes for this book, so it is not included in abundance here. It is used as a gelling agent, and is very useful for making raw desserts and pies. I recommend you check out the few recipes in the book and then go research some more; it is a wonderful ingredient to include in your diet, incredibly nutritious, and very useful when you want to make something a light and fluffy consistency.

Monatomic Trace Elements

The monatomic trace elements are a group of supplements that are found naturally occurring in volcanic soil, in the vicinity of Mount Shasta, California.

They are known as Etherium Gold, Etherium Pink, Etherium Black, and Etherium Red, and are produced by a company called Harmonic Innerprizes. The same company also produces a powder called Aulterra, which comes from an ancient seabed. The manufacturers describe them as "Supplements for the Spirit," and they work on a very subtle level, like a cross between trace mineral supplements and flower essences. They are vibrational remedies, restoring a lost balance within our very cells, our DNA. They contain substances that in ancient times would have been naturally occurring in the soil, but because of agricultural practices and intensive farming, we have lost these links to the earth. They have a powerful transformative effect on the user, enabling deep healing and shifts in stagnant energy. We have found them to be particularly powerful mixed in raw chocolate, where the essence of the supplement is carried right into the heart and mind in conjunction with the powerful healing vibration of cacao. This synergy seems to amplify and ground the effects, drawing it even deeper into the cells, and heightening the experience.

Mount Shasta is home to many spiritual communities. There have been many sightings of E.T.s and light beings there, and it is known for its otherworldly beauty and cloud formations. There are 28 conditions for the favorable building of a Buddhist monastery, and Mount Shasta is the only place in the world that fulfills every single one of them. The Etheriums were discovered in a meteorite crater in the vicinity of Mount Shasta. The meteorite was thought to have landed 5,000 years ago. So you could say these substances have literally been sent from outer space, to assist humanity in our transformation at this time. The Etheriums are the name given to the different strata in the soil deposits: Etherium Gold is the center of the crater, and then working outwards in rings are Etherium Red, Etherium Pink, and Etherium Black. Harmonic Innerprizes also produce other products, such as Shamir and Chamae rose. Shamir is about remembrance, similar to purple corn extract; it reconnects us with the ancient cellular memory, and the wisdom of our DNA. Chamae rose is a shrub that grows on the eastern side of the Sierra mountains, and assists in healing and detoxification.

The recommended dose for all these supplements is only ⅛ teaspoon, once or twice a day. Personally, as I am very sensitive, I notice the effects of a single dose of any of the monatomic trace elements instantly. I find they have a profound effect on my experience of the world. However, because they work on a very subtle level, many people who take them don't notice any difference at first. This is not to say that they aren't working, just that they are not noticing. I believe for people that have very deep-rooted issues, or who have certain aspects of their true selves very buried, they would still be having an effect on a subtle level which may take months to show up on the physical level. I would recommend taking one at a time to begin with. Etherium Gold is the best one to start with; if you are taking ⅛ teaspoon a day, a bottle will last you nearly two months. When When writing this book, I took Etherium Gold every day; it is excellent at helping us access our creativity. If I want to make a very special cake or chocolate, I will put them all in: this makes for an exceptionally magical day!

Etherium Gold has been scientifically proven to balance the two hemispheres of the brain. Humans spend too much time in our left brains, and not enough in our right brains; this imbalance is one of the major causative factors of discontent in our lives and in our societies. The left brain is concerned with the individual, the ego, survivalism, and linear, rational thinking. The right brain areas deal with community, oneness, bliss, and creative thinking. The left brain is limited and constricting, the right brain is infinite, expansive and abundant. So many problems in our cultures are due to excessive left-brain thinking, rather than thinking "outside the box," and seeing from the perspective that benefits the whole, the greater picture, rather than just the isolated self. Etherium Gold assists in correcting this imbalance, in restoring whole-brain thinking, "joining up the dots."

Etherium Gold contains traces of the minerals gold, iridium, chromium, silver, rhodium and platinum. It causes the body to produce more alpha brain waves. These are the ones that make us feel focused and creative. It reduces the levels of beta and theta brain waves, which are the ones we create when we are stressed. For this reason, taking Etherium Gold is like instant meditation. Users report greater levels of serenity and enhanced mental clarity when taking Etherium Gold; literally, it is helping us to achieve a higher state of consciousness. It helps with any sort of intellectual work: the three main foods that helped me write this book were cacao, Blue Manna and Etherium Gold. Cacao gave me the heart-centered energy to keep on with it every day; Blue Manna provided me with a sharp, clear, focused intelligence, and Etherium Gold kept me calm and creative. Two independent studies, one by the Alpha Learning Institute in Switzerland in 2003, the other by the Mind Spa in the U.S. in 1998, tested the brain waves using EEG (electroencephalogram) readings. In the Mind Spa study, the brainwave frequencies of 90% of respondents balanced out. "According to the Alpha Learning Institute, this level of focus and serenity in the brain is typically only observed in people who have either spent years practicing meditation or a martial art, engaged in months of light sound therapy, or taken seminars to train the brain for maximum performance. Yet, it was accomplished in just three days with Etherium Gold."

Etherium Gold is also said to assist with the manifestation of spirit into matter. Because of its electromagnetic pattern, the transformational process of energy into matter is accentuated, and the vibrational difference between thought and manifestation is reduced. This is why users report an increase in synchronicities and telepathic incidences once they start taking Etherium Gold —one of the most commonly reported side effects is an increased ability to find parking spaces! We gain mastery of our minds, and our ability grows to create the world around us as a true reflection of our hearts, rather than the distorted mirror of the ego.

There is currently growing international interest in the concept of Ormus. In the 1970s, David Hudson, a gold miner in Arizona, coined the term ORMEs, which stands for Orbitally Rearranged Monatomic Elements, when he discovered these strange materials on his land. Simply put, Ormus is precious metals such as gold, rhodium, iridium, silver and mercury molecularly arranged in a different state. It has been credited with having amazing healing properties and creating profound spiritual awakenings. Ormus is the elusive alchemical substance written about through history, in all different cultures. It is the holy grail, the Philosopher's Stone, the Elixir of Life, and taking it provides instant enlightenment. In the Bible, it is called manna, the Egyptians ate the Bread of the Presence of God, and the alchemical process of turning powder into gold features frequently in Hindu religious texts. The writer Sir Laurence Gardner links it with the Ark of the Covenant, and believes Moses made white powder into gold on Mount Sinai. Many of the superfoods are said to be rich in Ormus energy—goji berries, bee pollen, algae, maca, medicinal mushrooms, noni. I recommend taking some form of Ormus supplement regularly; as well as these superfoods you could consider specially formulated Ormus supplements such as Sunwarrior Ormus Supergreens and Shaman Shack Three Immortals. As a monatomic trace mineral, Etherium Gold has obvious links with Ormus, and understanding these helps shed light on some of Etherium Gold's amazing properties.

Aulterra rebalances and harmonizes the body's energy fields. It is a naturally occurring deposit taken from ancient seabeds, high in monatomic elements, which has been scientifically proven to activate and restore DNA. New age thinking has it that rather than just the two strands of DNA, we have 12. It is the ten hidden strands that contain encoded within them messages about our evolution, a higher consciousness. As we activate our DNA, we reconnect with the ancient wisdom of lost cultures, and also move forward into our divine consciousness. This is ascension, and it is what many of us believe humanity is going through now, at the beginning of the twenty-first century. Many people feel the changes in themselves, their bodies, their minds, their lives, but they do not know how to conceptualize that, and they do not understand how to integrate these different experiences into their lives. That is where these supplements come in, because they assist us in revealing our inner truths to ourselves, and then acting in accordance with them.

Our DNA is permanently oscillating, winding and unwinding. Aulterra resonates with the DNA molecule and causes changes to its structure that facilitates constancy in the oscillation. This constancy causes a quantum shift in the DNA, which produces light energy in the cells. Aulterra has been proven under scientific conditions to restore DNA, and act in a similar way to hands-on healing in restoring the body's life force. It has been demonstrated to provide protection against electromagnetic pollution, and is particularly beneficial to use when flying. It has also been demonstrated that Aulterra can improve the body's ability to utilize the nutrition within our foods. When many foods are lacking in the essential vitamins and minerals they once had, due to pollution and soil erosion, adding Aulterra to our foods can increase the amount of nutritional uptake we receive. As the recommended dose is only an eighth of a teaspoon, this is easily added to our foods. The Aulterra has to actually mix with the food to have the desired effect; it does not work if taken separately. Add Aulterra to each and every recipe in this book to really notice the power of Raw Magic!

Etherium Red integrates the thinking and feeling processes. It assists with clear decision-making, where we feel torn between our mind and emotions, or have to weigh up many different factors. By integrating the head and heart, stress is relieved and clarity is created. Etherium Red is also reputed to release the kundalini energy. Etherium Pink opens the heart chakra. It can help release issues of sorrow, grief and past hurt. It can be beneficial for people who are too much in their heads, and put them back into balance. When I take Etherium Pink, I feel as if I am in love with everyone! Etherium Black is about releasing blockages, it makes us feel grounded. It is an adaptogen, restoring homeostasis in the body and rebalancing the body's electromagnetic field.

Clearly, the monatomic trace elements are not a magical cure-all. It is not as easy as taking them and suddenly becoming realigned in body and mind, instantly transformed into a spiritually enlightened being. But they provide a doorway. At every moment in life we are making choices, consciously and very often unconsciously. We make decisions on what is possible, what is permissible, based on past experience, and very often these foundations are fear, hurt, judgment and loss. Taking the Etheriums keeps the other doorway open too, the doorway of love, joy, freedom and infinite possibility. Sometimes we cannot even see that doorway; sometimes we can see it but it seems too far away to step through. But it is massively helpful just to keep it open for when you are ready. This is why some people can take Etheriums and not notice any difference at first; it can take months before deep-set patterns are dissolved. When I first took Etherium Gold, it had no noticeable effect on me, and I didn't take it again for a couple of years. Now, I notice it instantly, because I am in the right place in my life to step through that doorway.

Hemp and Flax

"Wherever flaxseed becomes a regular food item among the people, there will be better health."
—MAHATMA GANDHI

"Make the most you can of the Indian hemp seed, and sow it everywhere."
—GEORGE WASHINGTON, HEMP FARMER

Hemp, flax and chia are the superfats. They are the only vegetable fats that contain all three of the Omega oils, the Essential Fatty Acids. EFAs are fats that the body cannot make, but which are essential for good health. The two major EFAs are omega-3 or -linoleic acid, and omega-6 or alpha-linolenic acid. You can also get EFAs from fish, but many people choose not to eat animals for ethical reasons, plus there are issues with the levels of toxicity in fish oils. EFAs work wonders for the brain, which is made of over 60% fat, and are excellent for the skin, as they increase the fluidity of the cell membrane. Studies have shown that taking EFAs on a daily basis improves brain function; for instance the Durham trial in the UK in 2002 demonstrated remarkable results for the one hundred school children who were given a fish oil supplement daily for six months. There was a noticeable improvement in concentration, learning ability, and behavior from the children who had the fish oil in contrast to the children who had the placebo. EFAs are also often used to treat skin problems like eczema and psoriasis, both as an external application in skin creams and oils, and when taken internally. They are a fantastic source of antioxidants, an essential nutrient for oxygenating the blood and preventing free radical damage. Other benefits associated with increased intake of EFAs include: an improvement in stamina and energy levels; a lowering of the risk of cardiovascular disease; metabolism balance and weight management; and an improvement in gut function.

In the West over the past few decades, a low-fat diet has been seen as a healthy diet. However, the tide of public opinion is beginning to turn, and people are realizing this is a misconception. The raw food diet is actually a relatively high-fat diet. Fats are essential to the body to metabolize foods, and if we are always starved of them, the body is permanently on alert, and so stores fat deposits in the cells, making the weight harder to shift. A diet abundant in healthy fats, however, means the body always feels nourished and so does not need to hoard excess fat in the same way. Fat nourishes the cell membranes and makes us shiny; healthy fats make us glow with inner radiance. Healthy fats include olives, avocados, nuts, and seeds (although, with the exception of coconuts, nuts should be eaten in moderation because they are mucus-forming and acidic).

Hemp contains omega-3, -6, and -9 oils in the perfect ratio for humans. Flax on the other hand has a higher proportion of omega-3s, which is the one that is harder to find in the diet, and the one most of us are lacking in. If you are new to these oils and are only going to take one, I would advise starting with flax to correct the balance in your body. But once you have upped your levels suitably, you can switch between either. Flax has a rich buttery flavor and a beautiful golden color; hemp is green and has a more distinctive nutty taste.

People often ask why can't they just eat the seeds since are so much cheaper than the pressed oils. Your body will extract some fats from the whole seed, but for most of us, our bodies are not working at their most efficient and will not be able to metabolize the seed effectively. EFAs are so important, and most of us are so depleted in them, I feel it is important to take the oil in its pure form and make sure the body is getting what it needs. So enjoy the whole seeds for their wonderful flavor as well as their nutritional content, in addition to taking the oil every day. Both hemp oil and flax oil are unstable, which means they go rancid easily and shouldn't be exposed to heat and light. Never cook with them! Buy only oils in dark glass jars and store them in the fridge.

Hemp is definitely in my top five most amazing foods on the planet. For a start, it loves Mother Gaia! It grows easily almost anywhere and is so hardy it needs no pesticides and chemicals, unlike cotton. Its growth as a crop nourishes the soil rather than depleting it, and benefits the environment by pulling carbon out of the air, making it the ideal food for sustainable farming. As well as being mega-nutritious, it is a great textile, makes beautiful paper, and is one of the best things you can put on your skin. THC, the psychoactive constituent in marijuana, is negligible in hemp grown for commercial uses. Most hemp comes from China or Canada. The hemp that is grown in Canada has the highest GLA content; hemp is the only plant source of gamma-linoleic acid.

Hemp seed comes in three forms: whole, shelled and protein powder. The whole seeds are a lot more nutritious because they have been left intact. (Though the whole seed may be impossible to find in the U.S.) When ground up and eaten fresh they are wonderful because the shells crack and the amazing properties of the oil are delivered straight to you. However, many people find the grittiness of the shells unpalatable. I like to use them in recipes in small amounts to add flavor and texture, but not solely as they can be overpowering. The shelled seeds are the seeds with their shells removed, and far more tasty and appealing, but will have lost some of their vitality and nutrients in the hulling process. They are small and white and soft, and much more popular, as they make wonderful smooth raw creams. Hemp protein powder is the seed with the fat extracted. This makes it exceptionally high in protein (48.5%). It has a deep earthy flavor, which goes equally well in sweet and savory dishes. I often add it to sauces and dressings for extra bulk, and it's commonly used in smoothies. Hemp protein powder is favored by athletes, and is also an excellent supplement for growing children. Hemp contains the full spectrum of amino acids, making it one of the few vegetables that is a complete protein, and furthermore the amino acids are in the perfect ratios for humans. It is also an excellent source of trace minerals, particularly magnesium. Add all this together and you have one of the most nutritional plants on the planet.

Flaxseeds or linseeds come from an herb that has also been popular historically as a fabric—this is where the name linen comes from. Flax oil is great used as a skin rub, to absorb the EFAs directly through the skin. I also always put flax or hemp oil into my enema water to get my EFAs direct through the colon wall. Flax oil has many health benefits: it has been shown to decrease blood pressure, it has anti-inflammatory and antiviral properties, and it enhances the immune system. Flax is a very strange seed, which acts unlike any others. It must be eaten either finely ground or soaked to receive

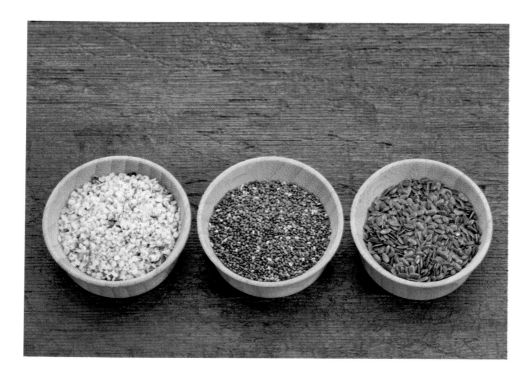

the health benefits. When it is milled, it should be eaten fresh before the oils start to decay. In this form, it acts as a thickening agent in recipes: one tablespoon of ground flaxseed mixed with three tablespoons of water is equivalent to one egg as a coagulant. It is often used in raw food cuisine as a binder for burgers and loaves. When soaked, they form a gloopy mass, a bit like frogspawn. They are not very palatable like this, but extremely health-giving, and a great digestive aid, acting as an intestinal broom, and helping with Irritable Bowel Syndrome. One cup of flaxseeds soaked overnight will absorb 3–4 cups water.

Chia is a South American seed that is new to most people, but is being adopted very rapidly by health-conscious individuals across Europe and the USA. It acts in a similar way to flax in that it swells up and absorbs up to four times the quantity of water. It's a popular breakfast porridge, a refreshing drink, or ground up in chocolates, cakes, crackers and burgers. The Mexicans consume it as *chia fresca*, by putting a spoon of chia and some lemon juice into a glass of water. The chia seeds will swell up within 15 minutes, and make a cleansing and delicious drink. Chia contains the highest amount of bioavailable omega-3 fats of any known plant food, and is also an excellent source of protein. It provides us with a clean, clear source of energy with no associated downside. The Mayans used it as fuel rations; they would march all day on as little as one to two tablespoons a day. It makes a great travel food because it absorbs up to four times its own volume in water, so a little goes a long way.

Coconut

The coconut is actually a fruit, growing mainly in southeast Asia.

It is a great source of protein, fats, vitamins and minerals, particularly potassium, calcium, sodium and magnesium. It is a really unique fat, and especially valuable to vegans and raw-fooders. When we start to cut out the denser foods from our diets like wheat and dairy products, we still crave heavier things to keep us grounded. The tendency is to reach for nuts, but they are fibrous and hard to digest. Too many nuts are mucus-forming, acidic and put the body out of balance. Coconuts on the other hand put less strain on the liver and pancreas, while still managing to get those denser fats into the diet. Coconut is one of the few plant sources of saturated fats. Coconuts have had bad press for a long time because it was assumed that all saturated fats were unhealthy, but the saturated fats in coconut do not raise cholesterol or contribute to heart disease.

The fats in coconut oil are medium-chain fatty acids, whereas most plant fats are long-chain fatty acids. Medium-chain fatty acids are burned up quickly in the body, but long-chain fatty acids get stored. Hence medium-chain fatty acids are a better source of energy and help with weight loss. Lauric acid is an essential fatty acid that is gaining wide recognition as being as important in the diet as the omega oils. Coconut is the only plant source of lauric acid, which has antiviral, antibacterial and antimicrobial properties. It can help the body deal with fungal infections, prevent viruses, and generally boost the immune system. Breast milk is the only substance that has a greater concentration of lauric acid. For that reason coconuts are considered a great thing to give to babies when they are weaning. When I drink coconut water, I imagine that's how breast milk must taste—sweet, nurturing, refreshing, energizing, calming, and balancing, all at once! Coconuts are similar in shape to a woman's breast, so I like to think of coconut water as nature's milk.

Coconut oil is also the only fat that is heat-stable, so it is perfect for cooking. All other fats oxidize when heated and become toxic to the body. Coconut is a great food for balancing the metabolism. Like cacao it seems to regulate the body's natural appetite and assist the body in maintaining its ideal weight.

It promotes healthy thyroid function and so can be very beneficial for people with both underactive and overactive thyroid conditions. There is evidence that it can help the body fight candida, IBS, Crohn's disease, diabetes, chronic fatigue, cancer, and HIV. Like hemp and flax, the coconut plant has a multitude of uses. The matting from the outer skin is known as coir and has a variety of uses such as in ropes, mats and brushes. The shells

- Young or jelly coconuts can often by found at festivals or Asian grocers, and are far superior to the brown ones in taste and nutrition. They are picked fresh off the coconut palm before they are fully ripe. To eat them, hack off the top with a machete or very sharp knife. Drink the water and scoop out the jelly-like flesh with a spoon, which is much thinner and softer than the brown nuts. A large

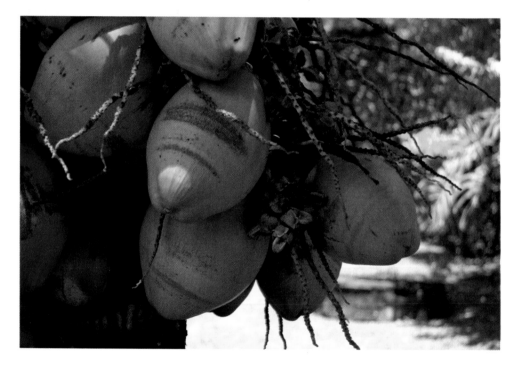

are made into household tools, drums and buttons. Coconut oil is one of the best things you can put on the skin and is popular as a natural lubricant.

There are many different ways to consume coconut. The best way is to travel to Asia and eat the fresh coconuts from the tree!

nut should provide around one liter of water. You can blend the flesh and water up together to make amazing raw coconut milk.

- Mature coconuts are the brown ones found in supermarkets. They have ripened, and fallen off the tree naturally. The flesh is much harder than that of young coconuts, and they contain less liquid. To eat, make a hole in the eyes with a screwdriver, and pour out the liquid into a glass. Then smash the coconut open with a hammer, and pry out the flesh with a knife or screwdriver. Wear gloves to protect your hands! Store the pieces in the fridge, and they'll keep for two or three days. We find they make a tasty and filling snack, instead of biscuits or sweets.

- Coconut butter/oil—the coconut oil market exploded in Europe and the USA in 2005 as news of its weight-loss and health-giving properties reached the mainstream. Note that coconut oil and butter are the same thing. In the UK it is more often butter and in the U.S. more commonly oil. Now there are many brands of good quality oil available. Look for those that are virgin cold-pressed. Since coconut oil melts at a temperature of 76°F, in cold weather it is solid, and in the summer it goes liquid. This property makes it perfect for sweet- and cake-making, because when melted it blends easily into other ingredients, and then can be hardened in the fridge to form solid sweets and cakes without cooking.

- Coconut water is popular as a sports drink because it balances the electrolytes in the body. You can buy coconut water in cartons ready to drink, but at the time of writing I am not aware of any brands that are raw. It is a brilliant source of minerals, vitamins and antioxidants. It is

fantastic after exercise or cycling. And as I've said, it's also a wonderful first drink for babies to help wean them off the breast.

- Coconut flakes are usually heat-treated to preserve them, so they are not technically raw. We use them in trail mixes, or sometimes blend them up to make a cream.

- Coconut milk commonly comes in tins and is made by blending the flesh and water and then is pasteurized to preserve it. It can be made at home, however, with fresh coconut.

- Desiccated and shredded coconut are the traditionally well-known forms of coconut, used as a cake and sweet decoration, but is rarely raw.

Coconuts are a part of my daily diet, and I find them to be a great source of clean energy. They satiate me without leaving me feeling heavy or dull, and are one of my main caloric sources of fuel. They give me a sustained and calm boost, particularly when combined with maca. We use them mostly in sweet- and cake-making, but also in sauces and puddings to add creaminess and richness.

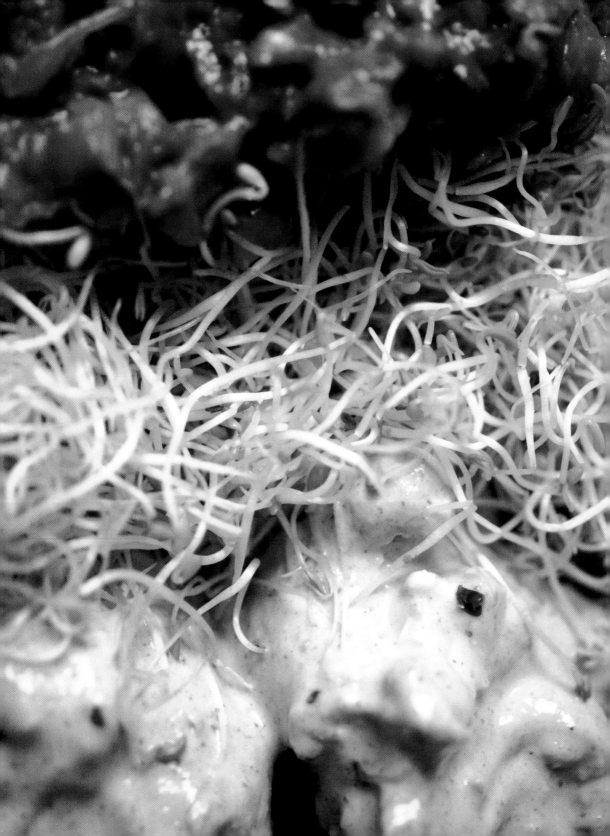

Recipes

I am so excited about superfoods in the kitchen.

I am a fervent believer that superfoods are not just for smoothies. These are FOODS, not supplements, and if you want to include them on a daily basis, I believe it is wise to integrate them into your existing menus rather than try and add new things in, which can cause confusion to your routine and overload your body. A sustainable healthy diet is one that is low in sugars, so I have invented tons of recipes to get your superfoods into your savory dishes. There are enough recipes here that you could eat chocolate every day without having any sugars at all! On the other hand, I have also included an abundance of sweet treats too. There are cakes, sweets and puddings galore, many of which contain more nutrition than the average square meal. This is not just healthy food, this is the best food ever! This food is so good, it is off the scale, in a class of its own. You can indulge yourself in the yummiest things you have ever eaten, you will not feel an ounce of suffering or denial, and you will have more energy and enthusiasm for life than you have ever had!

Grand claims? Try it for yourself—what have you got to lose? A few pounds, an annoying boyfriend, a job you don't like? This is the food of the revolution, food that will change your life, to give you the joy and vitality to make all your dreams come true. You might be saying, "Oh, I like my life, I am happy the way I am." Well, that's even more exciting. I liked my life before I started eating superfoods, I was really happy the way I was, I liked myself, my family, my friends, my work. But you know what? Since I started eating these foods daily, my world has shifted into a whole new orbit. Everything is possible, because I am the creator of my own reality, and the reality I am creating is so good. Eating superfoods helps us be the very best we can be, and every day just gets better. Life is an infinite and abundant path of reflection, inspiration, motivation, positive action, and integration. Ecstatic bliss becomes the norm. Shall I repeat that? Existence is ecstasy. Our natural state of being is to be as free as the birds, as wise as the horses, as rooted as the trees, as expansive as the mountains, and when we clear our lives of the clutter and debris which cloud our bodies and minds, we tune in to the majesty and beauty of the earth and reclaim the magic which is our birthright.

Every recipe in this book has been invented and tested and retested many, many times. So they definitely work! What's even better for you is that as this is the second edition of this book, we have had time to refine and improve on many of the recipes.

Chef's Notes

Buckwheaties

We use buckwheat a lot, in cereal, mixed into chocolate, and ground into flour for crusts and cakes. 300 g (2 cups buckwheat) makes 450 g (3 cups) buckwheaties. Put your buckwheat in a large bowl, cover it with water, and give it a good swish around. Drain it, then cover it in water again and leave it soaking for five hours, no more than eight hours max. Drain, and rinse once more. Leave it in the bowl to sprout for two or three days, giving it a rinse and a swish once a day. Once it's sprouted, with tails about the same size as the seed, no longer, spread it over drying trays (if you're using 300 g buckwheat this should spread over three trays). Dry for 12 hours. Stored in an airtight container, it will keep for a couple of months. My company, Raw Living, sells ready-made Buckwheaties, if you don't have the time or the resources to make your own.

Cacao Powder

Also known as chocolate powder, this is the cacao powder pressed direct from the bean, that hasn't been roasted or toasted. Conventional cocoa powders are always roasted and toasted.

Melting Butters

A lot of the recipes call for melted cacao butter and/or coconut oil. We've found the easiest way to do it is with a double boiler that heats food to controlled temperatures. If you don't have one, boil some water in a kettle or a pan. Then stand the butter in its jar in the pan, or transfer just what you need to a bowl, and stand that in the pan. Don't keep the water boiling, turn it off, or the butter will overheat. In warmer weather, you don't need to melt the coconut oil, it will be runny enough to use straight from the cupboard. If it's really hot, you don't need to melt the cacao butter either.

Salt

Crystal salt refers to any type of rock salt: sea salt, Himalayan salt, or any other natural mineral salt. When I travel, I like to pick up local interesting salts, such as Icelandic geothermal salt, Hawaiian red salt, or Indian black salt. Some of the recipes include tamari or miso as salt substitutes. I generally put a pinch of Himalayan crystal salt in everything I make, sweet or savory—it brings out the flavors and aids with the absorption of the minerals. Celtic sea salt is good too. I haven't put it in the recipes, but keep some on hand, because life is always best when taken with a pinch of salt.

Adding Water Gradually

When blending, it's vital to add the water gradually. If you pour it all in at the beginning of the recipe with all the other ingredients, it will not get amalgamated properly and the end result will be runny. Add the water slowly, a little by little: if you're using a cup of water (250 ml), add it a quarter of a cup at a time, blending as you go, and then your finished recipe will be the right thickness.

Weighing Avocados

An average avocado weighs 250 g, including the skin and stones, not just the flesh. Avocados vary a lot in size, so when a recipe calls for one or two, you may want to weigh them first to check how much you need. When a recipe uses a lot of avocado, it's usually safer going by weight than by counting avocados.

Etheriums

Where a recipe calls for one of the monatomic trace elements, this is for its energetic properties only and does not affect the taste. If you want to leave them out or substitute one for another, it's not going to affect the recipe working in the slightest, only the alchemical effects. The same goes for suma.

Sweeteners

In the book you'll find my preferred sweeteners. They are lucuma, mesquite, agave nectar, and xylitol. Lucuma is a powder made from a Peruvian fruit similar to a mango. It has a beautiful biscuitty flavor. Mesquite is another powder, made from a pod similar to carob. It has a sweeter, more caramelly flavor than carob. Agave nectar is a syrup made from the same cactus plant that tequila is extracted from. There has been some controversy surrounding agave nectar in recent years. I believe it's fine if you source it from a reputable manufacturer, and only use it in small amounts. Xylitol

is made from fermented birch bark, and it's a low-glycemic, healthy alternative to sugar. Some people are suspicious of it because it looks quite processed, but I have found a few spoonfuls in recipes is a great way to increase the sweetness without adding too much bulk. Not all brands of xylitol are raw, so check with the manufacturer if you want to be sure. Since I first wrote *Raw Magic*, coconut palm sugar has become another popular raw sweetener. Most brands are not raw; to my knowledge the Coconut Secrets brand is the only one that is. You can substitute xylitol for coconut sugar in any of my recipes, if you prefer.

Vegans

Strict vegans avoid the use of bee products. All the recipes in this book are vegan apart from those that include honey or bee pollen. Where honey is used, vegans can substitute agave nectar.

A Note on Superfoods

Since I wrote the first edition of this book in 2006, I have discovered many more "superfoods." I have come to feel that the term Superfoods is just a new way to describe what we have always known as herbal medicine. We are connecting to the natural healing power of plants, and I am confident that it's a journey that will never end, as we discover more and more about the magical way plants can interact with the human body. Some of the plants that I have discovered since the first edition of the book, I mention in the recipes: mushroom extracts such as reishi, Ayurvedic herbs such as ashwagandha, or one of my new favorite superfruits, baobab. Space does not permit me to go into detail on all of them here, or else this would turn into more of an apothecary handbook than a recipe book! But if this area of study interests you, please take time to keep up to date with our new discoveries by following my work online.

Equipment

There are a few basic pieces of equipment that I use time and time again for my recipes. If you have all of these in your kitchen, you'll be able to recreate everything in this book.

Blender
A really good blender is going to make all the difference to your ability to turn out fine raw cuisine. The Vitamix is the raw connoisseur's blender of choice; it's not cheap, but it does do everything—blend to within an inch of your life, and grind nuts and seeds to fine powders. If you haven't got a high-power blender, you need to be a bit inventive with a combination of a hand-held blender, a coffee grinder or spice mill attachment which comes with most blenders, and a food processor. And you still need a blender.

Dehydrator
If you're a raw-fooder, it's pretty likely that you'll have one of these already. They make raw crackers, biscuits, cookies and breads so good you'll never miss the cooked versions. If you don't have one, you can try using your oven on the lowest possible setting—the results aren't quite the same, but they're passable.

Double Boiler
We use this for melting coconut oil and cacao butter. If you don't have one you can use a saucepan and a Pyrex bowl that fits neatly inside it.

Cake Tins
Silicon molds are my preferred kitchen equipment for setting cakes, sweets, and chocolate. Not only does everything turn out easily, with a professional finish, everything sets quicker in silicon as well as it is a conductor of heat. If you don't have silicon molds, you can use a normal cake tin or baking tray, just line it with aluminum foil or baking parchment. You want a standard-sized tin or mold, somewhere between 7.5" (20 cm) – 9.5" (24 cm) in diameter. When you're making sweets, where I state medium-sized, the optimum is about 15 cm (6") square, and a large tray needs to be about half as big again (about 15 cm × 23 cm or 6" × 9".)

Cutlery
You need a couple of good tablespoons that you can always find when you need them, a heap of teaspoons, and a good ceramic chopping knife. Forks come in handy for digging coconut oil out of the jars and ground cacao nibs out of the bottom of the blender.

Measuring Cups
Apart from raw chocolate making, I measure just about everything using measuring cups. They are an essential element of your raw kitchen toolkit, alongside a ceramic knife, a nut milk bag, and a good selection of silicon molds. One cup is equivalent to 250 ml; weight-wise it varies according to what exactly you are measuring, e.g. one cup of almonds weighs more than one cup of coconut flakes.

Note on Tablespoons

The definition of a tablespoon differs depending what country you are in. In this book

One tablespoon = 3 teaspoons = 15 ml = 1/8 cup.

Big Fridge

Hell yeah. Preferably pink. Or silver. If it's white you need to cover it in stickers, magnets, and postcards.

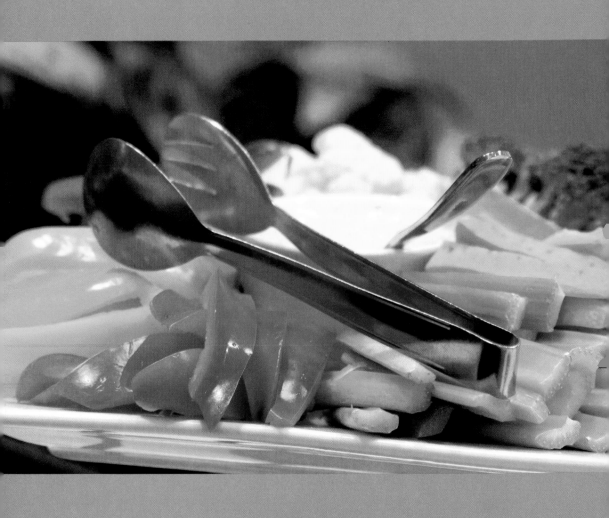

Dips and Dressings

Dips and dressings are central to raw food cuisine.

Having a selection of favorites in the fridge makes mealtimes easy and fast.

- Serve a dollop with crudités—don't just stick to carrots and celery, try red pepper, broccoli and cauliflower florets, fennel strips, zucchini sticks, endive leaves, turnip slices, daikon sticks, apple; be adventurous with your combinations and surprise your taste buds.

- Use in a wrap—nori sheets, cabbage leaves or romaine lettuce leaves make the best outer layers. If you're enthusiastic and you have a dehydrator, you can make lovely raw wraps with sprouted buckwheat or flaxseed. Stuff your wrap with pâté and sprouts, and munch away to your heart's content.

- Spread them on bread and crackers, raw or otherwise.

- Dips and pâté can be thinned out to make salad dressings. Add a little water or extra oil, get some good quality green leaves, preferably organic, local and seasonally grown, and voilà. A plate of rocket, half an avocado, a handful of sprouts, a sprinkle of cacao nibs, and a tasty dressing and you have a meal fit for royalty in less than minutes.

Most recipes given make enough for four to six servings, so you can make a batch, keep it in the fridge, and it should last you half a week.

You need a good blender to make most of these dishes. A standard store-bought blender will do the job, but for really professional results a high-speed blender is a fantastic investment. You can make do fine without one, but if you get one, you'll be really glad of it—it makes everything quicker, easier and tastier.

Cacaomole

Serves two
10 mins
Blender

This is one of my favorite lunches. Spread on a nori sheet and crammed with alfalfa sprouts, you couldn't fit any more nutrition in each bite. If you don't have a blender, you can still make this; just crush the garlic by hand, and mash everything up with a fork.

2 avocados
1 lemon, juiced
1 Tbsp hemp oil
1 clove garlic
1 tsp Seagreens or other sea vegetable granules
Pinch crystal salt
2 Tbsp cacao nibs

Remove the flesh from the avocados and place in a blender. Add the lemon juice, hemp oil, garlic, and Seagreens. Blend to a puree, adding water or more oil if you need to. Stir in the cacao by hand. Share it with someone who needs cheering up.

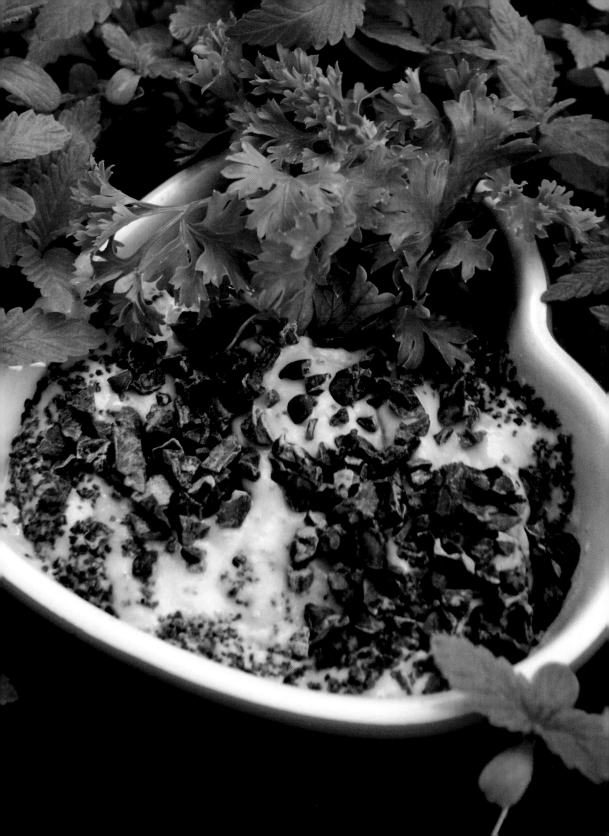

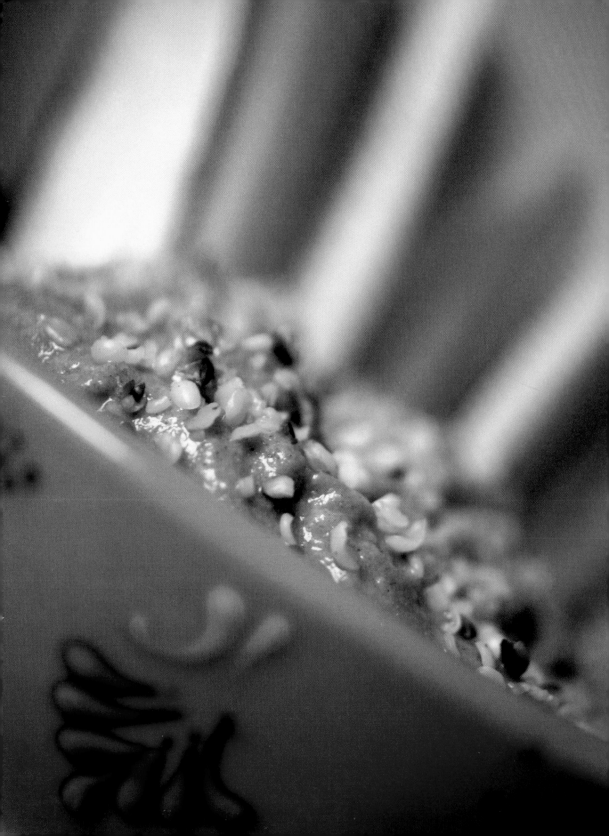

Hempamole

Serves four
10 mins
Blender

Having one of those days? Hempamole on Fire Wizard Crackers (p. 146) topped with alfalfa sprouts and a pinch of Crystal Manna will help you over any hump.

2 avocados
2 tomatoes
1 red chili
2 lemons, juiced
4 Tbsp hemp protein powder
1 clove garlic
1 tsp brown unpasteurized miso
2 Tbsp hemp oil
2 Tbsp shelled hemp seeds
1 Tbsp Seagreens or other sea vegetable granules

Remove the flesh from the avocados and put it in the blender. Remove the stems from the tomatoes, quarter them, and put them in the blender too. Remove the stalks and seeds from the chili and add that to the blender. Next add the lemon juice, hemp protein, garlic, miso and hemp oil and blend it all together to a thick cream. Stir in the hemp seeds and Seagreens by hand.

Bee's Knees Guacamole

Serves four
10 mins
Blender

Pollen and spices complement each other really well—this is guacamole with a sting. We buy organic vegan curry paste, but you can use whatever spicy seasoning you have in the cupboard.

2 avocados
2 tomatoes
2 Tbsp apple cider vinegar
1 clove garlic
2 tsp Thai vegan curry paste
1 cup (100 g) bee pollen
4 Tbsp dulse flakes

Remove the flesh from the avocados and put it in the blender. Quarter the tomatoes and add those in with the vinegar, garlic clove and curry paste. Blend to a thick cream. By hand, stir in the bee pollen and dulse flakes. Keeps in the fridge for up to a week, and actually improves after a day or two as the pollen starts to dissolve into the guacamole.

Crazy Carrot Relish

Serves four
10 mins
Grater

This is ridiculously good, as an accompaniment to a salad, or piled on top of crackers.

2 large (100 g) carrots, grated
¼ red onion
½ cup (50 g) bee pollen
2 Tbsp flax oil
1 tsp Thai vegan curry paste

Grate the carrot and transfer to a mixing bowl. Finely dice the onion, and put that in the bowl too. Add in the pollen, flax oil and curry paste and give it all a good stir together.

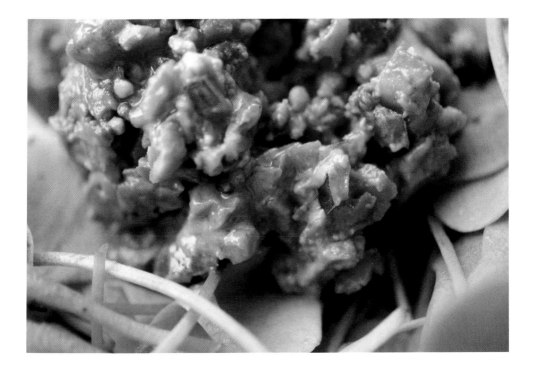

Greenvy

Serves four
10 mins
Blender

Like gravy but green, I love this dip for its apple-like shade and delicate flavor. Shelled sesame is not so nutritious as the whole seed, but it makes a much tastier cream. Use as a dip for crudités, or add a little water to thin and use as an alkalizing dressing for green salad leaves.

- 1 cup (125 g) shelled sesame seeds
- 1 Tbsp cold-pressed, extra-virgin olive oil
- 1 Tbsp apple cider vinegar
- 2 Tbsp barleygrass powder
- ½ tsp crystal salt
- 1 cup (250 ml) water

Put all the ingredients together in the blender with half the water. Add the rest of the water gradually while the blender is running, and blend for a few minutes until it makes a thick cream. Will keep in the fridge for up to a week.

Greyvy

Serves 8
10 mins
Blender

Like greenvy, but grey. We use this as a gravy for green vegetables like broccoli, peas, and sauerkraut. It's so tasty, you can pour it liberally over your veg for a satisfying quick meal.

- 1 cup (125 g) hemp seeds, shelled
- 2 Tbsp raw tahini
- 4 Tbsp hemp protein
- 1 Tbsp liquid aminos
- 1 Tbsp kelp granules
- ¼ tsp Chaga extract or other mushroom powder
- 4 Tbsp hemp oil
- 1 cup (250 ml) water

Put all the ingredients in the blender, with half the water. Blend to a cream, so that the hemp seeds are completely amalgamated. Add the rest of the water gradually, with the blender running until it reaches the desired consistency. Will thicken a little if left in the fridge.

Chocolate Mayonnaise

Serves four
10 mins
Blender

Wow! I don't know what else to say. Just, wow. Use as a dip, or thin for a dressing. Goes great on seaweeds.

2 cups (250 g) shelled hemp seed
½ cup (50 g) cacao nibs
1 Tbsp raw tamari
1 Tbsp cold-pressed, extra-virgin olive oil
1 lemon, juiced
1 clove garlic
1 cup (250 ml) water

Put all the ingredients in the blender with half the water. Blend to a thick cream, then add the rest of the water gradually with the blender running until you have a thick dollopy consistency.

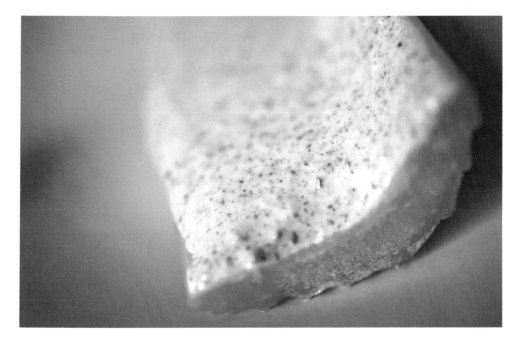

Cranberry and Goji Relish

Serves four
10 mins
Blender

Perfect at Christmas or Thanksgiving with your Omega Love Loaf (p. 147) and Cacaoslaw (p. 111).

3 tomatoes
1 cup (100 g) fresh cranberries
½ cup (50 g) goji berries
½ cup (50 g) dried cranberries
¼ onion
½ chili
1 tsp apple cider vinegar

Put everything in the blender and blend for a few minutes. Will thicken when left in the fridge.

Goji Ketchup

Serves eight
10 mins, presoaking 30 mins
Blender

This is so popular, a sweet tangy relish, which is perfect for children. Usually we just eat it as it is, with some green crudités like broccoli, cucumber and celery.

3 large tomatoes
1 cup (100 g) gojis
½ cup (50 g) sun-dried tomatoes, soaked 30 mins
¼ red onion
1 Tbsp cold-pressed, extra virgin olive oil
1 Tbsp apple cider vinegar
1 tsp tamari

Soak the tomatoes for 30 minutes in the purest water available. When they're ready, drain them, and put everything in the blender together. Blend for a couple of minutes, until you have a smooth puree. Keeps well for up to a week in the fridge.

Greatest Garlic Goji Relish

Serves eight
10 mins
Blender

Everyone adores this, especially children. It's one of my most popular dips, with an amazing fruity flavor you know is filling your cells with fun.

  1 whole (200 g) sweet red pepper
  1 cup (100 g) goji berries
  2 Tbsp apple cider vinegar
  2 cloves garlic
  ½ tsp salt

Chop the red pepper into pieces big enough for your blender, carefully removing all the seeds. Put everything in the blender together and blend until the gojis are mashed and there's no bits left. Keeps in the fridge for up to a week.

Broccoli Bonkers

Serves four
10 mins
Blender

> This is a greener-than-green dip for when life gets a bit too bonkers and you need reassuring that at least your dinner makes sense, if nothing else.

1 small (250 g) head broccoli
¼ red onion
2 Tbsp spirulina
2 Tbsp cold-pressed, extra virgin olive oil
2 lemons, juiced
1 Tbsp nutritional yeast flakes
1 Tbsp raw tahini
1 Tbsp Seagreens or other sea vegetable granules

Chop the broccoli into small pieces to fit into your blender. Put all the ingredients apart from the Seagreens into the blender together, and give it a good going until it's creamy. If it's too much like hard work for your blender, you can add a little water in or some extra oil. Once it's turning over and there's no lumps of broccoli left, stir in the Seagreens by hand. Keeps for a few days, or you can dehydrate leftovers and crumble them into croutons for salad.

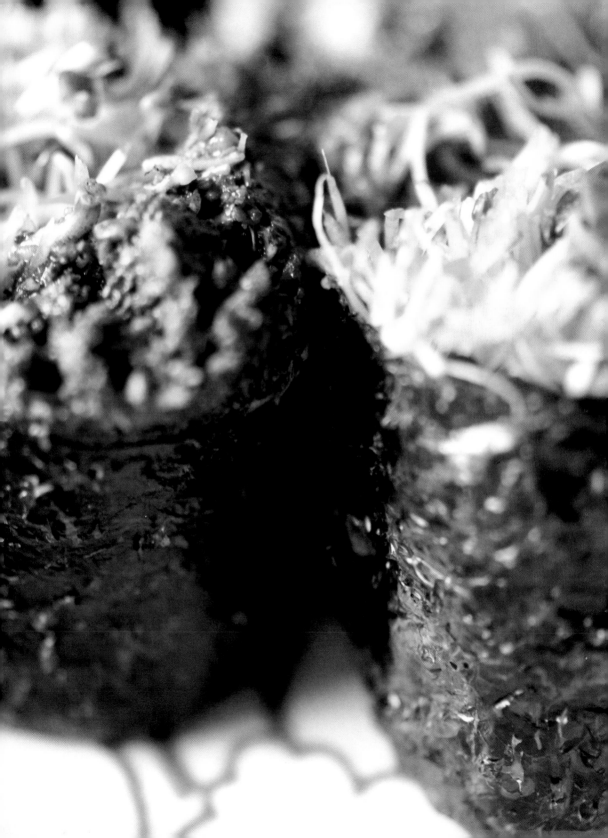

Spread It On Your Bread

Serves four
5 mins
No equipment needed

We love tahini on our bread, but too much of it is heavy on the liver, and mucus-forming. So we add lemon juice to create more of a balance. When you mix lemon juice into tahini, it has a thickening effect, so you also need to add a lot of water. This way, you're making your tahini go twice as far! Aulterra increases the absorption of nutrients in the food: we often add it to salads and dips.

2 Tbsp raw tahini
1 lemon, juiced
2 tsp brown unpasteurized miso
1 Tbsp flax oil
½ tsp Aulterra
4 Tbsp water

Put everything but the water in a small bowl and mix together with a teaspoon. When you have a thick paste, add the water, a spoon at a time, until you reach the desired consistency.

Purple Pesto

Serves eight
10 mins
Blender

This pesto is such a beautiful color, gorgeous spread thinly on crackers, or use as salad dressing for some purple leaves like oakleaf or radicchio.

1 large bunch basil
¾ cup (100 g) shelled hemp seeds
1 clove garlic
2 Tbsp cold-pressed, extra-virgin olive oil
2 Tbsp apple cider vinegar
1 Tbsp agave nectar
1 tsp purple corn extract powder
1 tsp white miso

Prepare the basil for the blender. You can use most of it; you may want to discard some of the ends if they are very thick and woody. Put everything in the blender together, and blend until you have a gorgeous thick paste.

Magic Maca Pesto

Serves four
5 mins
Blender

Maca works equally well in savory and sweet dishes, adding an interesting flavor and energizing your food. This works as a dip or a dressing.

1 large bunch basil
1 cup (100 g) sesame seeds
½ cup (50 g) maca
4 Tbsp hemp oil
1 Tbsp agave nectar
1 Tbsp apple cider vinegar
1 Tbsp tamari
1 clove garlic

Prepare the basil for the blender, removing any exceptionally thick stems. Put everything in the blender together with half the water and blend to a paste. Add the rest of the water gradually while the blender turns, until you have a thick cream. Eat within 24 hours as maca doesn't keep well.

Many Ways Mayonnaise

Serves eight
10 mins
Blender

This is a perfect staple to keep in the fridge for dipping, dressing, spreading, dehydrating, spooning, licking, sucking—now I'm just getting carried away.

1 ¾ cups (200 g) shelled hemp seeds
½ cup (50 g) maca
1 tsp Aulterra
¼ tsp crystal salt
2 Tbsp cold-pressed, extra-virgin olive oil
2 lemons, juiced
1 clove garlic
1 cup (250 ml) water

Put everything in the blender together, apart from the water. Blend together for a minute, then add the water gradually while the blender is turning. Keep in the fridge—doesn't keep well, eat within a few days.

Mayo Maynot

Serves four
10 mins, 3 hours setting
Blender

This has all that over-richness of traditional mayonnaise that makes you want to dip fries in it and forget about your thighs in a few moments of unmeasured ecstasy. However, because as we all know by now, coconut oil balances your metabolism and so doesn't make you put on weight, you can eat this safe in the knowledge that you can have both unmeasured ecstasy and divine thighs.

1 cup (100 g) coconut oil
2 Tbsp brown unpasteurized miso
3 lemon, juiced
½ cup (100 g) raw tahini
½ cup (125 ml) water

If you're in a cold climate, the coconut oil will be hard, and you need to melt it in a heatproof bowl over a pan of freshly boiled water. If it's hot where you are, then the coconut oil will be soft and you don't need to heat it, you can just blend it as it is. Blend everything together. Leave in the fridge to set, although you can eat it as it is, warm and dribbly.

Macand of Dressing

Serves four
5 mins
No equipment needed

This is my kind of dressing, simple but decadent. It makes a beautifully easy dinner poured over a pile of green leaves like arugula, baby leaf spinach and lamb's lettuce.

1 Tbsp raw tahini
2 Tbsp hemp oil
1 Tbsp maca powder
1 tsp white miso
½ lemon, juiced
¼ cup (60 ml) water

Put all the ingredients apart from the water into a small bowl. Gradually pour in the water, stirring as you add it. Once you have a creamy thin sauce, it is ready. You can store leftovers in the fridge, but maca doesn't keep well once mixed with water; eat within a few days.

Gardner Street Dressing

Serves four
10 mins
No equipment needed

When we had the Raw Magic shop in Brighton, my friend Alex and I used to go to Infinity wholefoods and buy greens and avocado. Then we'd hide behind the counter and make this in paper cups with plastic spoons, mix it all up in a big bowl with some Sunseeds and cacao nibs out of the pick 'n' mix, and feed each other. A customer would come in and we'd sit there with purple and green mouths, trying to look all innocent. Which we're both quite good at.

2 Tbsp barleygrass powder
1 Tbsp raw tahini
1 Tbsp flax oil
1 lemon, juiced
½ tsp crystal salt
½ tsp purple corn extract
4 Tbsp water

Put everything in a bowl (or a paper cup) apart from the water. Stir it with a spoon until it's evenly mixed. It looks a bit of a boring brown colour but taste it and you'll be amazed at how lively it is. Add the water gradually until you reach the desired consistency for your dressing.

Manitoba Dressing

Serves four
10 mins
Blender

This is another one of those super ideas to have hiding in the fridge, ready to do exciting things with when you get in at 7:00 and haven't got many brain cells left. Pour it over leaves, grated carrot, finely chopped broccoli, anything and everything that's loitering in your fridge drawers and hey presto, instant dinner manifestation. It's named after Manitoba Harvest, Canada's leading hemp heroes.

1 cup (125 g) shelled hemp seeds
½ cup (125 ml) cold-pressed, extra-virgin olive oil
2 Tbsp brown rice vinegar
2 Tbsp hemp, coconut or liquid aminos

Put everything in the blender and keep going for a minute or so until it's creamy. If you can't be bothered to blend the sauce, you can omit the hemp seeds and just make a vinaigrette.

Finest Flax

Serves six
10 mins
Blender

> You're best off using this dressing straightaway—if it sits in the fridge, the flax-seeds will swell and absorb the oil so it's more gloopy. When it goes like this, just give it a good stir and maybe blend in some extra lemon juice and water if you want it runnier, although I like it the way it is; it coats the salad in a kind of clumpy fashion.

½ cup (75 g) flaxseeds, ground
½ cup (125 ml) flax oil
½ tsp crystal salt
2 lemons, juiced

Grind the flax in a coffee mill or high-power blender. Put everything together in the blender and blend until you've got a gloop, baby.

Salads and Savories

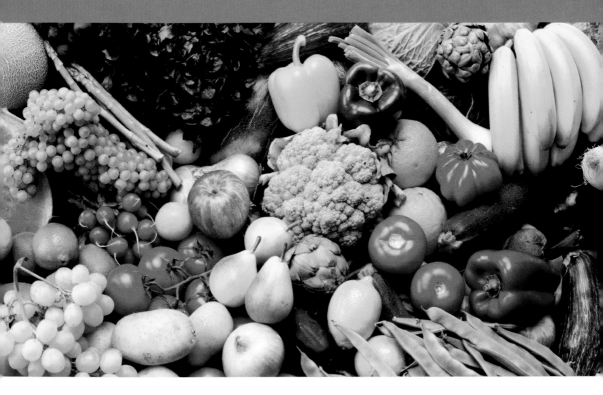

In case you hadn't got the message by now, I am truly passionate about getting you to put superfoods in your dinner. I think it's important that we use them as any other kitchen ingredient, like vegetables and herbs, rather than reserving them for special occasions or only putting them into sweets and smoothies. They shouldn't be considered as supplements, they are foods, and if we want to really experience the benefits, we need to integrate them into our existing menus and make sure we get plenty every day, at every meal. This is a whole new way of eating that will bring an unparalleled dimension of pleasure to your mealtimes. Start eating the Raw Magic way and life will never be the same again.

Cauliflower Cream

Serves four
10 mins, 3 hours presoaking
Blender

Soothing and nurturing, kind of like mashed potato. If you try it and you don't like it, or you've got some leftovers, you can spread it onto dehydrator trays—it makes good crackers.

½ cup (75 g) flaxseeds, presoaked
¾ cup (200 ml) water
½ (200 g) cauliflower
2 Tbsp raw tahini
2 lemons, juiced
2 tsp brown unpasteurized miso
1 clove garlic
1 tsp kelp powder

Presoak the flaxseeds in the water for at least three hours. They will absorb all or most of the water—don't throw any away. Put the cauliflower, tahini, lemon juice, miso, garlic and kelp in the blender with the flaxseeds and blend to a smooth cream. After a minute or two, once there's no lumps of cauliflower left, it's ready. Eat the same day—cauliflower doesn't keep well once blended.

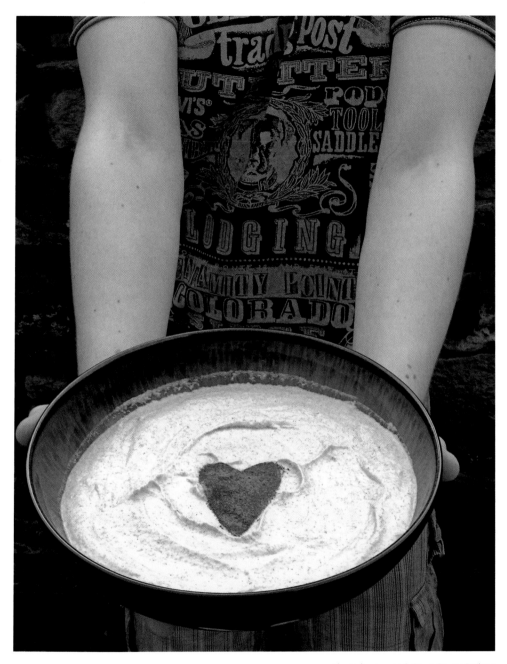

Photo by James & Dewi Druce-Perkins

Naughty Noodles

Serves four
20 mins
Spiralizer or grater

> A spiralizer is the raw-fooder's favorite gadget for making raw noodles and pasta. It's inexpensive, easy to use, and fun to play with. If you haven't got one, you can grate the squash instead; it's not the same effect but it still works.

    1 medium-sized butternut squash
    4 Tbsp cacao powder
    2 Tbsp raw tahini
    2 Tbsp hemp oil
    1 tsp chili powder
    1 lemon, juiced
    1 Tbsp tamari
    ¼ cup (60 ml) water
    2 Tbsp cacao nibs
    2 Tbsp shelled hemp seeds
    4 Tbsp dulse flakes

Cut your squash into eight pieces, in half across the middle and the two halves into quarters lengthways. Scoop the seeds out of the bottom half. Place each piece in the spiralizer with the noodle setting on, or grate using a food processor. Transfer your noodles to a large mixing bowl. In a smaller bowl, blend the cacao powder, tahini, hemp oil, chili powder, lemon juice, tamari and water, using a spoon. You should have quite a runny dressing. Pour this over the noodles with the nibs, hemp seeds, and dulse flakes. Give it all a good mix together so the dressing is evenly covering the noodles and there are no clumps left. Serve with a green salad and Macand of Dressing (p. 98) or Supersexy Curry (p. 115).

Jonny's Luminous Soup

Serves two
Blender
10 mins

I read a lovely quote that said, "We have the ability to develop the luminous energy fields of angels within this lifetime." It became a running joke with my friend Jonny and me—"I can't come to the phone, I'm just developing my luminous energy field...I've forgotten what I was saying, I got distracted by developing my luminous energy field," that kind of thing. So this is Jonny's Luminous Soup, specially designed to help you develop your very own luminous energy field.

2 stalks celery
1 cucumber
1 cup (50 g) spinach
1 (250 g) avocado
2 Tbsp hemp oil
1 lemon, juiced
2 cups (200 g) broccoli florets
1 clove garlic
2 Tbsp shelled hemp seeds
2 Tbsp barleygrass powder
½ tsp Crystal Manna or E3 AFA flakes

Prepare the celery, cucumber, spinach and avocado for your blender by removing unwanted stems etc., and chopping them small enough that they won't cause trouble for your machine. Put them all in, along with the hemp oil and lemon juice. Blend to a liquid. Then add in the broccoli, garlic, hemp seed and barleygrass powder and blend again until you have a cream. Serve by warming gently, and garnish each bowl of soup with ¼ teaspoon Crystal Manna flakes.

The Ultimalkalizer Soup

Serves two
Blender
10 mins

> This soup contains everything you need to alkalize and energize—all that cucumber, a generous serving of barleygrass and a sprinkling of nori flakes.

1 ½ cucumbers
¾ cup (100 g) shelled hemp seeds
1 Tbsp apple cider vinegar
½ tsp crystal salt
1 Tbsp barleygrass powder
1 Tbsp maca
1 Tbsp nori flakes

Chop the cucumbers into pieces that will go into your blender happily. Put them in with the hemp seeds, vinegar and salt, and give it a good blend until you have a liquid with no chunks of cucumber or bits of hemp seed left. Add the barleygrass and maca and give it another quick whiz. Warm gently if you like, and serve sprinkled with nori flakes.

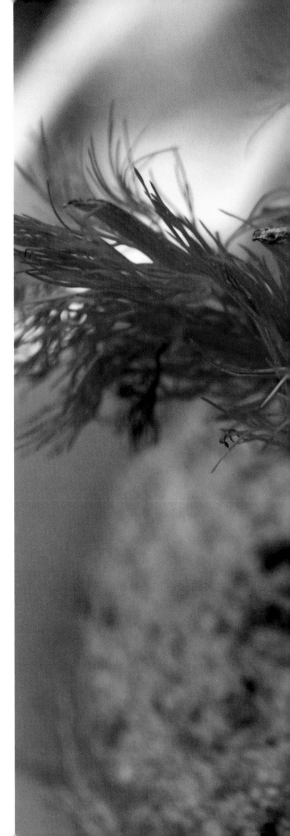

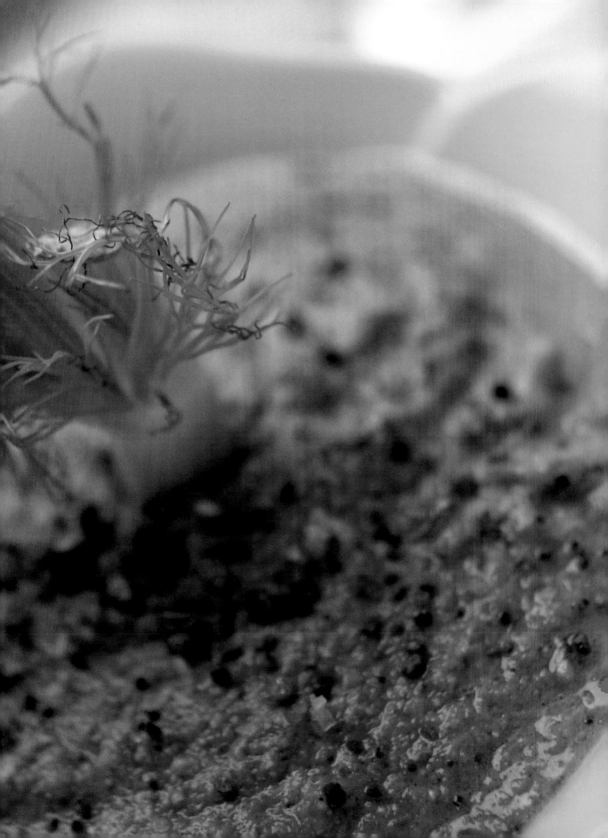

Tonya's Tasty Chocolate Cream

Serves two
Blender
15 mins

This sauce is lovely served warm, to release the aromatic oils of the cacao. Pour over a mix of your favorite vegetables like spinach, cauliflower, and steamed butternut squash. I've named it after Tonya Kay, one of the most committed and inspiring raw vegans I am blessed to know.

¾ cup (100 g) cacao butter
2 large tomatoes
1 yellow pepper
4 stalks celery
¾ cup (100 g) shelled hemp seed
1 clove garlic
1 Tbsp agave nectar
½ tsp crystal salt

Start by melting the cacao butter. While it is melting, prepare your tomatoes, pepper and celery for the blender by removing extraneous stalks, stems and seeds and chopping them into pieces small enough not to worry your blender. Blend the vegetables up to a liquid. Then add in the hemp, garlic, agave nectar, salt and melted butter and blend again.

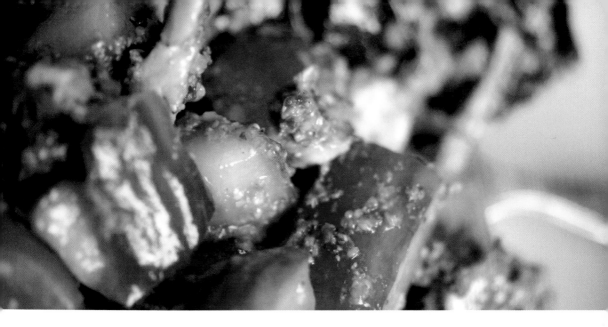

Crystal Cumber Number

Serves two
No equipment needed
10 mins

Ooh baby, I've got your number. This dish is the epitome of what I am trying to convey with these dinners: impressively quick and easy, inexpensive, and so nutritious you could live on it.

3 Tbsp flaxseed, ground
2 avocados
1 cucumber
1 tsp Seagreens or other sea vegetable granules
1 tsp Crystal Manna or E3 AFA flakes
1 Tbsp flax oil
pinch crystal salt

Grind your flaxseeds if you haven't done so already. Cube the avocados into bite-sized pieces and spoon out the flesh into a mixing bowl. Cube the cucumber into pieces the same size and add them to the bowl. Stir in the Seagreens, Crystal Manna, flaxseed, flax oil and crystal salt. Make sure it's evenly mixed, and serve as a light lunch or tea.

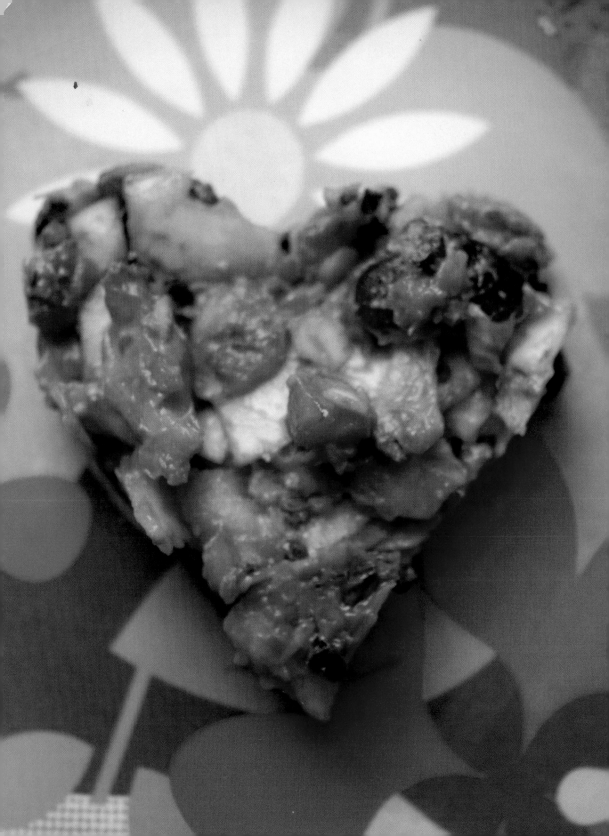

Cacaoslaw

Serves four
15 mins
Food processor, blender

Adding a sprinkle of cacao nibs to any salad lifts it to a whole new level. Coleslaw is such a basic it can become boring, but as you may have noticed by now, eat enough superfoods and the word "boring" starts to disappear from your vocabulary.

2 carrots
1 apple
½ red onion
2 cups (200 g) white cabbage
2 avocados
1 Tbsp apple cider vinegar
pinch salt
1 clove garlic
1 tsp purple corn extract
½ cup (125 ml) water
½ cup (75 g) cacao nibs

Top and tail the carrots. Quarter the apples and remove the core. Finely grate the carrots, apple, onion, and cabbage. To make the mayonnaise, blend the avocados, vinegar, salt, garlic, purple corn extract and water. Toss the vegetables in the mayonnaise, along with the nibs. This salad will keep for a day or two, as the vegetables soften and the flavors deepen.

Bold Barleygrass Stew

Serves one
No equipment needed
10 mins

This is a lovely warming winter dish, so simple to make, but very nurturing and satisfying.

½ red pepper
¼ head broccoli
1 stalk celery
1 Tbsp bean (mung or mixed) sprouts
1 Tbsp corn kernels
2 Tbsp dulse flakes
2 Tbsp flaxseeds, ground
1 Tbsp barleygrass powder
1 tsp brown unpasteurized miso
1 cup (250 ml) water, boiled
¼ tsp chili or curry powder
¼ tsp Cordyceps or other mushroom extract

Prepare your pepper, broccoli and celery by chopping them into small bite-sized chunks, a little bigger than the corn kernels. Grind the flaxseeds if they are not already pre-ground. Put the seeds in a bowl with the barleygrass, miso, and chili or curry powder, and add the water a little at a time, stirring gently. Add more water if you want a thinner, less gloopy stew. Once you have added in the water, stir in the vegetables and all the remaining ingredients. Eat at once while it is warm. If you have a double saucepan, you can make this by putting all the ingredients in the pan, and heating it up that way.

Macauliflower Cheese

Serves four
15 mins, 12 hours presoaking
Blender

This is a beautiful rich cheesy cream that is so good it might not actually make it onto the cauliflower. Don't worry if it doesn't, make some Many Ways Mayonnaise (p. 97) as well and use that instead.

1 cup (125 g) cashews, soaked 8–12 hours
1 (500 g) cauliflower, divided into bite-sized florets
1 lemon, juiced
1 tsp white miso
2 Tbsp nutritional yeast flakes
2 Tbsp maca
1 cup (250 ml) water

Presoak the cashews overnight. Put the cashews, lemon juice, miso, nutritional yeast flakes and half the water in the blender and blend for a minute until there are no lumps of cashew left. Add in the maca, and as the blender is turning, add the rest of the water gradually. Chop the cauliflower into large bite-sized pieces, trying to preserve the florets as much as possible. Pour the sauce over the cauliflower, toss and serve. If you would like it warmed, you could spread it over a dehydrator tray, heat it for 4–6 hours, and serve straight from the dehydrator. Eat within a day or two; cauliflower doesn't keep well.

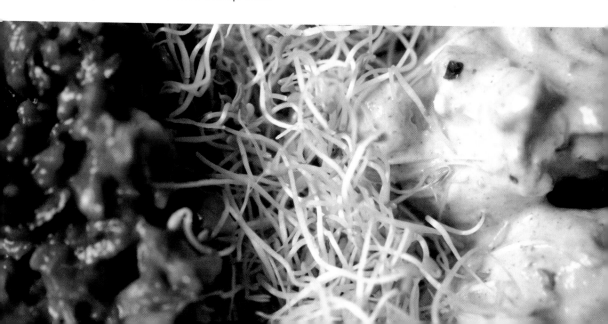

The Orange Orgasm

Serves four
Blender
15 mins

If you make this for a potential lover, and he doesn't hoist you over his arm in a fireman's lift and carry you straight to the bedroom, then it's definitely time to give up, girls, and start looking around at some of the other fish in the sea.

¾ cup (100 g) cacao nibs
¾ cup (100 g) shelled hemp seeds
¾ cup (100 g) coconut oil
3 tomatoes
2 red peppers
½ red onion
1 red chili pepper
½ cup (50 g) goji berries
2 Tbsp dulse or dulse flakes
2 tsp tamari
1 tsp suma powder
¼ tsp Reishi or other mushroom extract

Grind the nibs, hemp and coconut oil together in the blender until you have a thick granular cream. Prepare the tomatoes, pepper, onion and chili pepper for the blender. Make sure you remove all the seeds from the chili pepper. Pop them in the blender with the goji berries, dulse, tamari and suma and blend again. Keep blending for a couple of minutes until you have a smooth orange cream. Serve accompanied by a green salad.

Supersexy Curry

Serves one
15 mins
Blender

Charged with superfoods, this dinner is perfect for feeding to your very own god or goddess.

1 large avocado
3 small tomatoes
2 stalks celery
¼ red onion
1 lemon, juiced
2 Tbsp shelled hemp seeds
2 tsp curry powder
1 Tbsp maca powder
¼ tsp suma powder
1 cup (100 g) cauliflower
½ red pepper
1 cup (50 g) spinach
1 Tbsp goji berries

Peel and pit the avocado, and put the flesh into the blender. Halve the tomatoes, and chop the celery sticks into eighths, and put them in the blender too. Add the onion, lemon juice, hemp seeds and curry powder and blend to a thick puree. Add in the maca and suma and blend briefly. If you blend maca for too long it goes bitter. Remove the sauce from the blender and put in a bowl. Chop your cauliflower into small bite-sized pieces, and dice your pepper into pieces the same size. Stir the cauliflower, pepper, spinach and gojis into the sauce. Eat straightaway.

Christal Kale

Serves four
No equipment needed
5 mins, 2 hours marinating

The really dark, leafy green vegetables like kale, spinach and chard are about the best vegetables you can eat, especially when they're in season and locally grown. However, they can be quite fibrous and chewy to eat just as they are raw, so raw-fooders often use a technique called wilting, as described here. The presence of the oil also helps with the digestion of the kale. This is Chris' favorite, so I named it after him.

8 cups (400 g) kale
3 Tbsp cold-pressed, extra-virgin olive oil
½ tsp crystal salt
2 avocados
4 Tbsp dulse flakes
2 Tbsp shelled hemp seeds
1 cup (100 g) Raw Living Sunseeds*
2 tsp Crystal Manna or E3 AFA flakes

Chop the kale into small bite-sized pieces with a good knife, and transfer to a mixing bowl. Pour the olive oil over and sprinkle in the salt. With your hands, give the kale a good massage. Really rub the oil and salt right into the leaves. This will soften and tenderize them and make them more palatable. Massage the kale for a couple of minutes, then cube the avocado and add that into the mix with the dulse flakes, hemp seeds, Sunseeds (if you can't get Sunseeds, you can just use a mixture of pumpkin and sunflower seeds), and one teaspoon Crystal Manna. Give it all a good mix in, and transfer to a large serving dish. Sprinkle the second teaspoon of Crystal Manna over the top evenly, then leave in the fridge for at least two hours to marinate. This dish keeps well for a couple of days.

*Can be purchased at rawliving.eu. Shipping to the U.S. is surprisingly affordable.

Balance Your Hempispheres Salad

Serves two
No equipment needed
10 mins

If you can't get enough of hemp, this is the salad for you. Hemp comes to us in many forms, and this salad contains just about all of them. Serve with some hemp burgers (p. 153) and Hempilicious Ice Cream (p. 174) for pudding and you'll be transported to hempiven.

1 cup (50 g) arugula
1 cup (50 g) baby leaf spinach
1 cup (50 g) lamb's lettuce
1 cup (50 g) alfalfa sprouts
1 cup (100 g) sauerkraut
2 Tbsp cacao nibs
4 Tbsp shelled hemp seeds
4 Tbsp whole hemp seeds (if available)
2 Tbsp hemp protein
1 avocado
2 Tbsp hemp butter
1 Tbsp hemp oil
2 tsp liquid aminos
1 lemon, juiced

Put the arugula, spinach, lambs lettuce, alfalfa, sauerkraut, cacao, hemp seeds (both types), and hemp protein in a salad bowl together. Cube the avocado flesh and add it to the salad. Give it all a good mix, so the sauerkraut and alfalfa are evenly threaded, not in clumps. In a small separate bowl, mix the hemp butter, hemp oil, liquid aminos and lemon juice with a spoon. You should have a runny paste to pour over your salad. As you toss the dressing in the salad, it will clump together into a dense mix. Serve immediately.

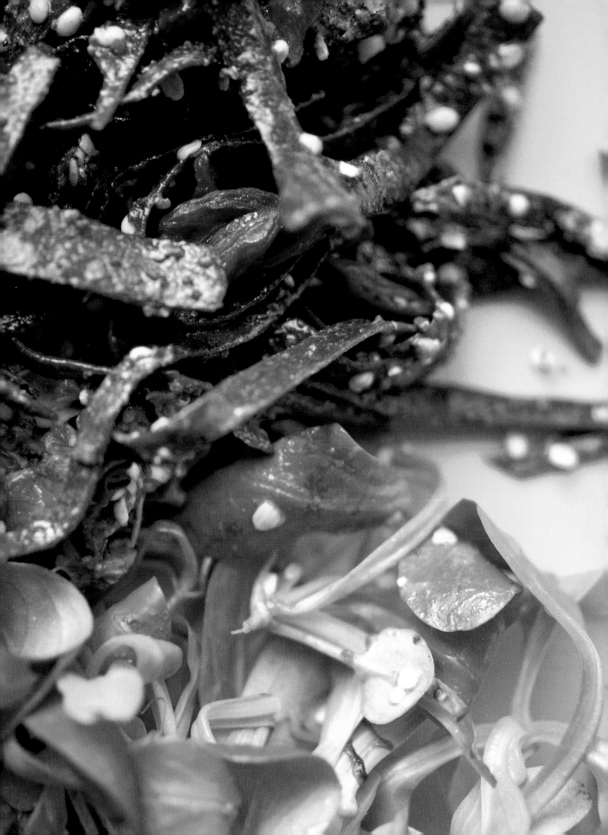

Spaghetti Gojous

Serves four
No equipment needed
5 mins, 30 mins or more presoaking

The fruitiness of the gojis complements the saltiness of the spaghetti really well in this dish. In Chinese cuisine, gojis are often used in chicken or duck dishes, and it is easy to see why once you start adding them into your dinners.

140 g (or sheet 25 cm × 25 cm) sea spaghetti, presoaked at least 30 mins
4 Tbsp goji berries
4 Tbsp shelled sesame seeds
1 tsp kelp powder
1 Tbsp apple cider vinegar
4 Tbsp cold-pressed, extra-virgin olive oil
½ tsp crystal salt

Presoak the sea spaghetti for at least 30 mins, but preferably overnight. When it's ready, drain, and stir in all the other ingredients and it's ready to serve. Will keep in the fridge for up to a week.

Sky-High Spaghetti

Serves four
5 mins, 30 mins or more presoaking
No equipment needed

My friend Sky loves seaweed and he loves hemp, so this recipe was named after him. Hemp and seaweed are one of my favorite combinations, really grounding, calming and rebalancing.

140 g (or sheet 25 cm × 25 cm) sea spaghetti, presoaked 30 mins
1 cup (50 g) alfalfa sprouts
2 Tbsp shelled hemp seeds
2 Tbsp hemp protein powder
2 Tbsp hemp oil
1 Tbsp Seagreens or other sea vegetable granules
2 tsp liquid aminos

Presoak the sea spaghetti for at least 30 mins, but the longer the better as far as this seaweed is concerned. When it's ready, drain and add all the other ingredients to the bowl. Give it a good stir and it's ready to serve. Will keep in the fridge for up to a week.

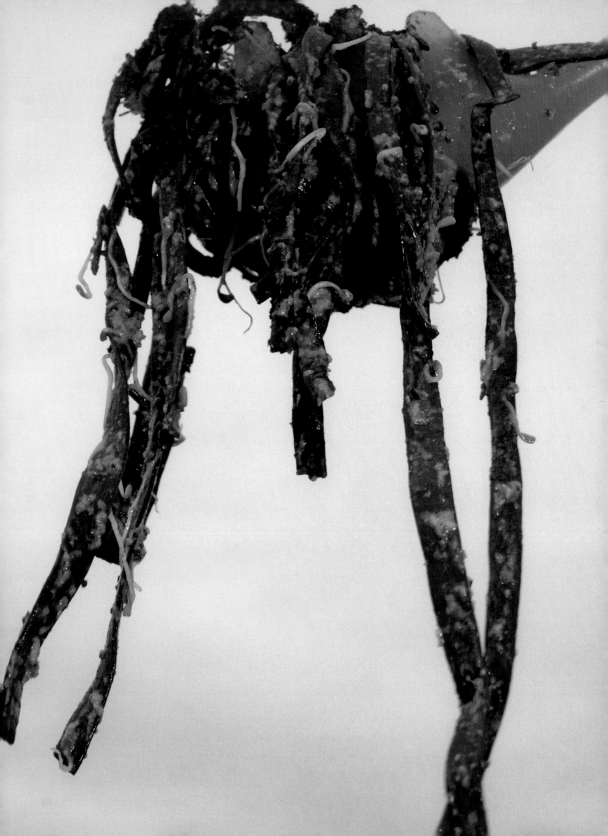

Multidimensional Sea Vegetable Salad

Serves four
5 mins, 20 mins or more presoaking
No equipment needed

Take a mix of any of your favorite sea vegetables. We favor dulse, wakame, sea lettuce, and sea spaghetti. Use as many different varieties as you can get your hands on, and then add your yummiest simple dressing to it, for a meal fit for Neptune, made with no fuss or drama.

25 g mixed sea vegetables, presoaked for the required time
4 Tbsp flaxseeds, ground
2 Tbsp nutritional yeast flakes
1 Tbsp balsamic vinegar
2 Tbsp sesame oil
2 tsp tamari

Presoak the sea salad for at least 20 minutes. It needs a lot of water, at least four times the quantity of water to sea salad. If you haven't got pre-ground flaxseeds, grind them now. When the seaweed is ready, drain, and add all the ingredients to the bowl. Give it a good toss, and it's ready to serve. Keeps well in the fridge for up to a week.

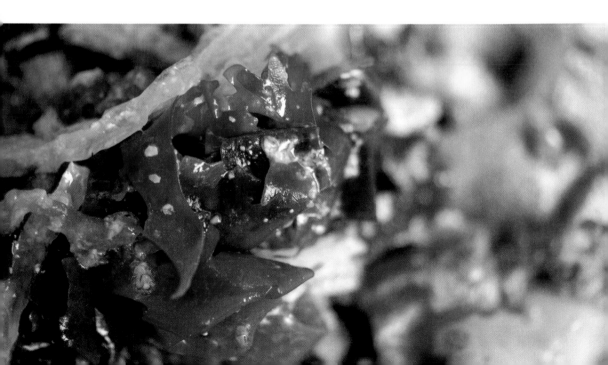

Wild Spaghetti Western

Serves four
10 mins, 30 mins or more presoaking
No equipment needed

Wild foods are really good to include in your diet—they keep you in touch with your natural instincts, and are full of nutrition because they haven't been intensively farmed. Herbs are close to wild foods, especially those that are organically grown.

140 g (or sheet 25 cm × 25 cm) sea spaghetti, presoaked 30 mins
2 avocados
1 large (100 g) bunch parsley
2 Tbsp maca
2 Tbsp hemp protein
1 cup (100 g) sauerkraut

Presoak the spaghetti for at least 30 minutes, but preferably overnight. Drain it when it's ready. Cube the avocado flesh and add to the seaweed. Chop the parsley as fine as you can, and add that too. Add the remaining ingredients and give it all a good mix together. Eat on the same day, or the maca starts to go bitter.

Rockin' Broccoli Salad

Serves two
15 mins
No equipment needed

A good salad, unlike a good man, isn't hard to find. Take something green, something from the sea, an avocado, something sprouting and something fermenting, and drown them in dressing; there you have my basic rules for assembling magic meals in minutes. Of course, you don't need to use every one of those elements every time. This salad uses four out of the five and shows you how it's done.

1 cup (50 g) dulse
2 avocados
1 cup (100 g) broccoli
½ cup (25 g) alfalfa sprouts
3 Tbsp flaxseeds
2 Tbsp hemp oil
½ tsp salt
1 tsp purple corn extract
½ lemon, juiced
½ tsp chili powder

Rinse the dulse and put it in a large bowl. Halve the avocadoes, remove the stones, cube the flesh, and spoon it out into a bowl. Fine-chop the broccoli into bite-sized pieces. Add all the remaining ingredients to the bowl and give it a good mix with a spoon.

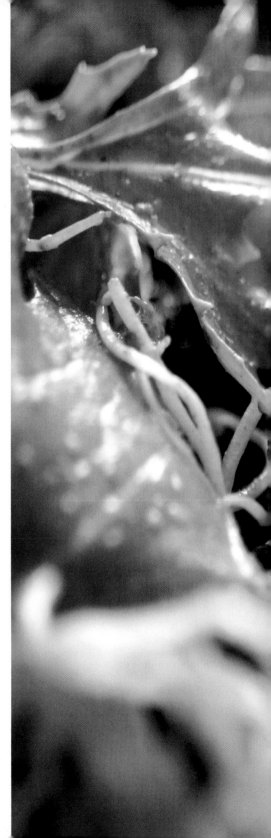

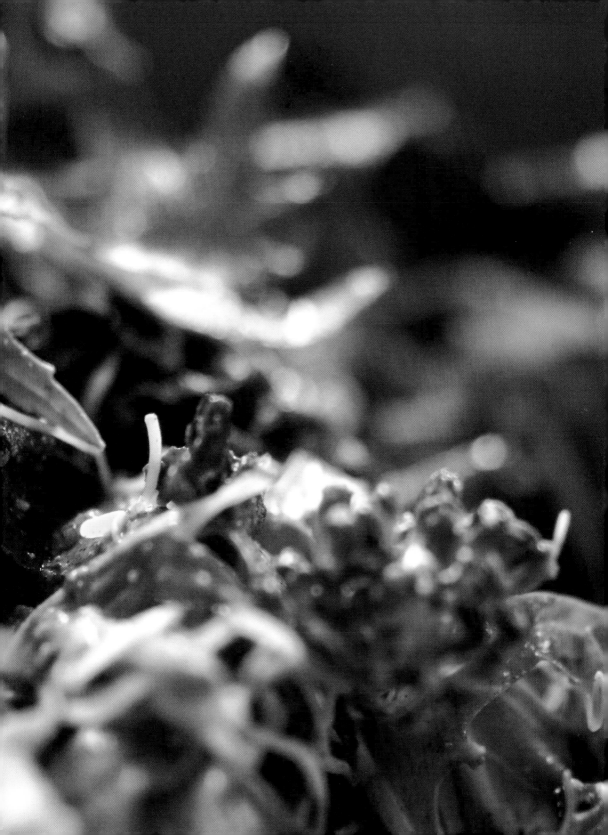

Ecstatic Being Salad

Serves two as a main course or four as a side dish
No equipment needed
10 mins

This has everything in it—seaweed, hemp, cacao, maca, barleygrass, algae, gojis, reishi. Eat it every day for guaranteed enlightenment.

1 large purple oakleaf lettuce
½ cucumber
2 avocados
½ red onion
Small bunch cilantro
½ cup (25 g) dulse
1 cup (50 g) alfalfa sprouts
2 Tbsp shelled hemp seeds
2 tsp Seagreens or other sea vegetable granules
4 Tbsp cacao nibs
½ cup (50 g) Sunseeds*
2 Tbsp goji berries
4 Tbsp Greenvy (p. 90)
2 Tbsp maca
1 tsp Crystal Manna or E3 AFA flakes
¼ tsp Reishi extract

Tear the lettuce into bite-sized pieces. Rinse in a salad spinner for best results. Transfer to the salad bowl. Finely slice the cucumber and add to the salad bowl. Cube the avocado, and add. Dice the red onion as small as possible, and chop the coriander finely, add these in too. Rinse the dulse and add that in. Add the alfalfa sprouts, hemp seeds, Seagreens, cacao nibs, Sunseeds, goji berries and maca, and give it all a good toss so it is evenly mixed. Add the Greenvy, and toss again, making sure the dressing is evenly coating the salad. Divide between the serving plates, and sprinkle with a little Crystal Manna for garnish. Bliss!

*www.rawliving.eu

Sweet and Spicy Sunshine Soup

Serves one
10 mins
Blender

> Guaranteed to lift your spirits on a gloomy winter's day. This soup loves you and it wants you to be happy.

2 tomatoes
1 red pepper
2 carrots
2 stalks celery
1 avocado
1 red chili pepper
1 clove garlic
1 lemon, juiced
1 cup (100 g) gojis plus a few extra for garnish
¼ tsp crystal salt

Prepare your tomatoes, pepper, carrots, celery, avocado, chili and garlic for the blender, removing any unwanted seeds and stems, and cutting into pieces small enough not to overload your machine. Put in the softer foods at the bottom, like tomatoes and pepper; carrots and celery are more likely to get stuck in the blades and jam it up. Add in the lemon juice and gojis, and blend for a few minutes until you have a thick gloop. You can warm this gently in a double saucepan, or just eat as it is. Garnish with a handful of gojis and a splattering of crystal salt.

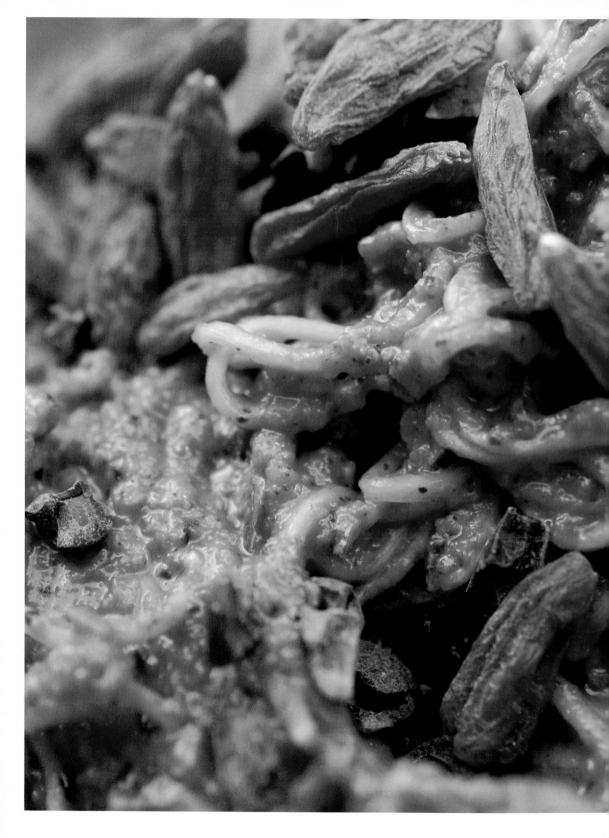

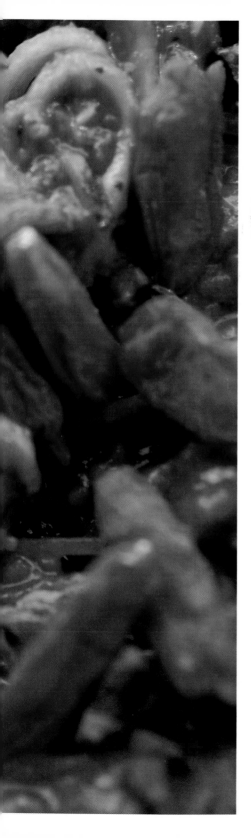

Go Go Goji Sauce

Serves two
15 mins
Blender

This is a version of my eternally variable Pasta Sauce recipe which crops up in my books, magazine articles, workshops and has even appeared on TV a few times. Basically, it is a simple recipe which you can alter in an infinite multitude of ways to create something different every time. Here it is chock-full of gojis for a super fruity sauce. Pour over veggies, steamed or raw, or add to wheat-free pasta, rice or quinoa.

3 tomatoes
1 carrot
2 stalks celery
¼ red onion
1 avocado
1 cup (50 g) dulse
1 cup (100 g) goji berries
1 Tbsp cold-pressed, extra-virgin
   olive oil
1 Tbsp apple cider vinegar
1 tsp tamari

Prepare your tomatoes, carrot, celery, onion and avocado for the blender by removing unwanted seeds and stems, and cutting into pieces to fit your blender without it complaining. Put them all in, along with the remaining ingredients, and give it all a good whiz for a few minutes until everything has amalgamated. Will keep in the fridge for up to five days.

Cacao'd Up
Marinara Sauce

Serves four
15 mins
Blender

Pasta sauce again, this time with chocolate. Inevitable, really. The presence of fats and sugars actually slows down the action of cacao in the body, so putting it into savory dishes like this gives you a purer cacao buzz, and should mean you end up eating less.

⅓ cup (50 g) cacao nibs
⅓ cup (50 g) cacao butter
5 tomatoes
4 stalks celery
2 carrots
1 avocado
2 cloves garlic
1 large bunch basil
1 Tbsp apple cider vinegar
½ tsp salt
4 dates

Pre-grind the cacao nibs in a grinder or high-speed blender. Grate the cacao butter, and put it in the blender with the ground nibs. Remove the stalks from the tomatoes and quarter them, put them in the blender. Roughly chop the celery and carrots so they're easy for the blender and pop them in too. Scoop out the avocado flesh with a spoon and in it goes. Next goes the garlic, basil, vinegar, salt and dates. Blend for a few minutes. You may find the cacao butter goes a bit lumpy, that's OK. Remove the sauce from the blender and either put it in a double saucepan, or in a Pyrex bowl sat inside a saucepan of hot water. Heat the water until the sauce is very slightly warmed and the butter is melted in. It's gorgeous to eat it warm like this.

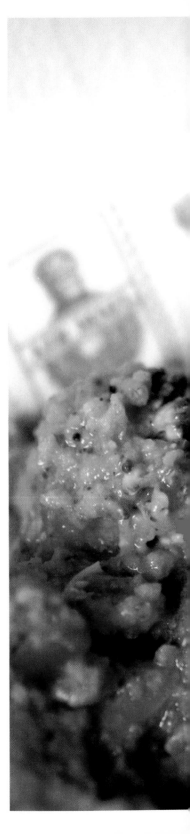

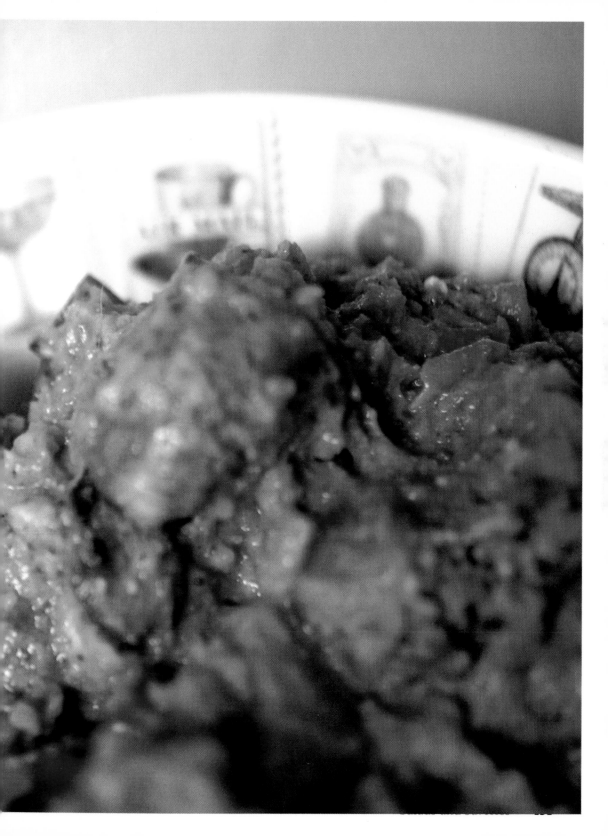

Polly's Perfect Nori Rolls

Makes 2 rolls
5 mins
No equipment needed

This is even better if you use the fresh bee pollen, rather than the dried kind.

2 nori sheets
1 Tbsp almond butter (white, if available)
1 tsp white miso
1 Tbsp flax oil
1 Tbsp apple cider vinegar
2 Tbsp bee pollen
½ of one avocado
2–4 broccoli florets
Handful or two of baby leaf spinach
4 Tbsp alfalfa sprouts

Lay out the nori sheets. In a small bowl, mix up the almond butter, miso, flax oil, vinegar and bee pollen with a teaspoon. Spread half of the mixture on each nori sheet, as a line along the middle lengthways. Half the avocado, and cube the flesh. Put half an avocado in each sheet, over the almond butter mix. Cut the broccoli into small bite-sized pieces, and put half in each sheet. Next lay out the spinach and the alfalfa sprouts along the sheet, next to the avocado. With a little water on each sheet, wet the edges of the sheets' lengths; this will help it stick together when you roll it. Roll them up, rolling the edge nearest you over first, keeping it tight. Press the far edge down. If they're just for you, eat them as they are, like a baguette. If you're serving them to friends or family, you can cut each roll into four and stand them on end on a plate—they look very pretty this way.

Rocket Fuel Soup

Serves two
15 mins
Blender

This has a spicy kick that will shift you up a gear. Makes a brilliant fast lunch. Heat it in the winter or have it chilled in the summer.

2 tomatoes
2 peppers
4 stalks celery
1 avocado
1 red chili pepper
2 cups (100 g) arugula
1 cup (50 g) dulse
3 Tbsp cacao nibs

Prepare your tomatoes, peppers, celery, avocado, chili and arugula for the blender by removing any seeds and stems and cutting them into manageable pieces. Rinse the dulse, and put all your ingredients in the blender together, setting aside one tablespoon cacao nibs. Whiz away for a few minutes until you have pureed everything until it's smooooooooth. Garnish with the remaining nibs.

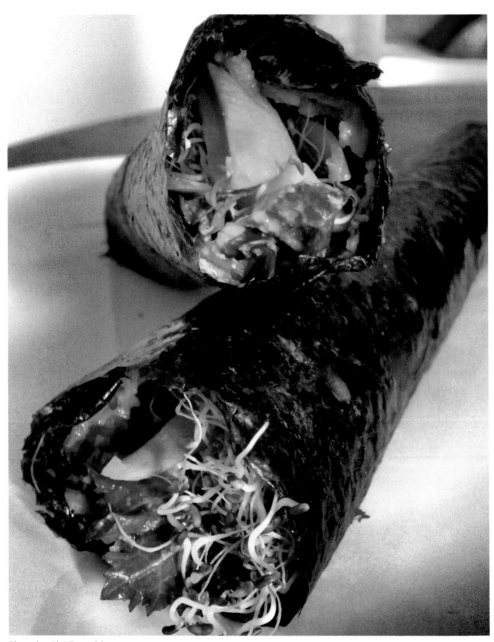

Photo by Alej Reynolds

Rawlicious Roll-Ups

Makes four rolls
10 mins
No equipment needed

I find this the perfect dinner on the move, it fills me up and gives me energy to keep going with the next thing, happy and contented.

4 nori sheets
2 Tbsp raw tahini
1 Tbsp hemp oil
1 lemon, juiced
¼ tsp crystal salt
1 tsp Crystal Manna or E3 AFA flakes
½ tsp Blue Manna or E3 AFA Mend
1 large carrot
¼ cucumber
4 leaves lettuce
Alfalfa sprouts

Lay out your nori sheets. In a small bowl, mix up the tahini, flax oil, lemon juice, crystal salt, Crystal Manna, and Blue Manna with a spoon. Spread this mix in your nori rolls, half in each roll, in a wide strip lengthways across the middle of the roll. Cut the carrot and cucumber into thin matchsticks, and lay these over the spread, half in each roll. Then tear the lettuce into small pieces, and put two leaves in each roll. Finally, add the alfalfa, laying it alongside the vegetables. Wet the long edges of the nori sheet and roll tightly, starting with the end nearest you. Press the far edge down, and it's ready to eat. If you've made them for yourself, I would just eat them like that, it's more satisfying. If they're for sharing, slice each roll into quarters with a sharp knife, and serve standing up on a plate so you can see the spiral patterns inside the roll.

Magic MultiColored Kale

Serves two
20 mins
Blender

> This makes an amazing purple, green and red salad with three
> of my favorite salad ingredients: seaweed, greens and cacao.

25 g Clearspring (or other brand) Japanese sea vegetable
  salad
3 cups (150 g) purple kale (or green kale if you can't find it)
2 Tbsp cacao nibs
1 tbsp Seagreens or other sea vegetable granules
2 Tbsp shelled hemp seeds
1 avocado
1 Tbsp apple cider vinegar
1 tsp agave nectar
1 clove garlic
1 tsp tamari
1 small bunch basil
1 tomato
1 tsp purple corn extract

Soak the Japanese sea salad in plenty of water, at least four times
water to seaweed. While you're waiting, you can prepare the
other parts of the dish. Take the kale and slice it into bite-sized
slivers. Put it in the salad bowl with the cacao nibs, Seagreens and
hemp seeds. Remove the flesh from the avocado and put it in the
blender—we are going to make an avocado pesto similar to the
one in my book *Raw Living*. Put the vinegar, agave nectar, garlic
and tamari in the blender. Remove excess stems from the basil and
chop loosely. Quarter the tomato, pop it in the blender with the
basil, and give it all a blend together so you get a thick cream with
no bits of basil left. When it's ready, transfer to the bowl with the
kale in. By this time your sea salad should be ready; drain and add
that to the bowl too. Give everything a good mix together, sprinkle
with purple corn extract, and it's ready to eat.

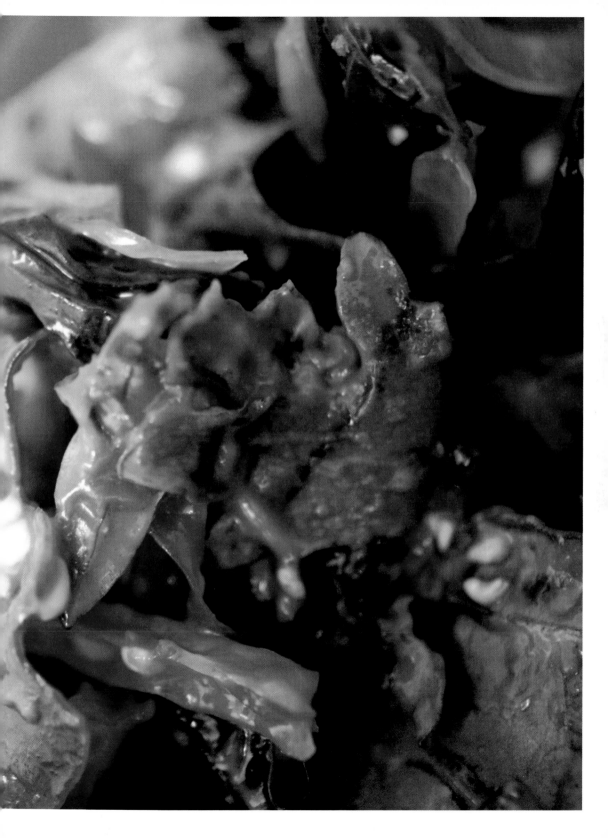

Ani's Thai Curry

Serves four
15 mins, 12 hours presoaking
Blender

> If I'm in a hurry, I like to cheat and use ready-made curry pastes. They're not raw, but the flavor is professional and authentic and it's so much quicker and easier than trying to track down Oriental herbs. There are many good organic, vegan, sugar-free ones on the market; try a few and discover your own favorite brand. This one is named after my gorgeous friend Ani Phyo, who is at the cutting edge of raw vegan Asian fusion cuisine.

½ cup (60 g) almonds, soaked 12 hours
1 cup (60 g) sun-dried tomatoes, soaked 1 hour
1 cup (100 g) goji berries, soaked 1 hour
3 tomatoes
2 carrots
2 red peppers
4 stalks celery
½ red onion
1 bunch cilantro
1 Tbsp Thai vegan curry paste
2 Tbsp cold-pressed, extra-virgin olive oil
1 lemon, juiced
1 cup (100 g) broccoli
1 cup (100 g) cauliflower
1 red pepper
1 cup (50 g) spinach
½ cup (50 g) cashew nuts

Presoak the almonds overnight. Soak the tomatoes and gojis one hour in advance. If you soak them separately, you can drink the goji soak water, I love it. Prepare your tomatoes, carrots, one of the red peppers, celery, onion and cilantro for the blender by removing unwanted seeds and stems and chopping into small pieces so that they will not be too much hard work for your machine. Put the veg in the blender with the drained almonds, tomatoes and gojis, curry paste, olive oil and lemon juice. Whiz away for a few minutes until you have a thick puree. Remove from the blender and transfer to a large bowl. Prepare the broccoli, cauliflower and the remaining red pepper by dicing into small bite-sized pieces, removing unwanted seeds from the pepper. Add them into your sauce, along with the spinach and cashew nuts and give it all a really good stir, until the sauce is evenly coating the veg, and it's ready to go.

Hot Rockin' Chia

Serves four
Takes 10 minutes to make and 2–3 hours to marinate
No equipment needed

Chia dinners are my new favorite thing! Perfect for meals on the run, I make a big bowlful the night before a busy day and leave it marinating overnight. I get three really good meals out of this, and you could easily stretch it to four. If I'm super busy it serves as lunch AND dinner. Otherwise it keeps in the fridge for about five days and actually improves with age. I like to make this with garlic-infused olive oil and the results are outstanding.

    1 cup (150 g) chia seeds
    4 cups (1 liter) water
    2 Tbsp cold-pressed, extra-virgin olive oil
    2 tsp raw vegan pesto
    ½ tsp asafoetida
    1 tsp Crystal Manna or E3 AFA flakes
    1 avocado
    1 cup (20 g) kale pieces
    ½ cup (25 g) sunflower salad greens

Soak the chia in four cups (one liter) water. You can add in all your other ingredients at the same time: the oil, pesto, asafoetida and crystal manna can be stirred in as they are. The avocado needs to be chopped into bite-sized pieces and stirred in. The kale needs to be torn into tiny pieces first. It doesn't really wilt in the chia unless you leave it for a few days so you may want to wilt it first by massaging it with olive oil and salt, before you stir it in. I love sunflower salad greens; if you don't grow them yourself, you can buy them from whole-food stores, they are usually kept with the alfalfa. If you can't get hold of any, substitute with your favorite sprout or green vegetable.

Give it all a really good stir and then leave it for at least three hours, until the chia has absorbed all the water. It doesn't need to be left in the fridge. If you can give it a quick stir now and then while it's marinating, all the better. Serve as it is for an instant meal, or with a side salad to make it into a proper dinner.

Chocolate Curry

Serves two
15 mins, 12 hours presoaking
Blender

Cacao and spices are a natural combination, and this green curry will have you wondering why we don't traditionally put chocolate in savory foods more often, it works so well.

1 cup (125 g) almonds, soaked 12 hours
½ cup (60 g) cacao nibs
2 Tbsp hemp oil
1 cup (50 g) spinach
4 stalks celery
2 tomatoes
1 avocado
½ red onion
½ tsp crystal salt
2 tsp curry powder

Presoak the almonds overnight. When they're ready, drain, and add to the blender with the cacao nibs and hemp oil. Prepare your veg for the blender by removing unwanted stems and seeds and chopping them into small pieces that won't block up the blender. Put everything in, and give it a good whiz for a few minutes until you have a thick puree. Serve as it is, or stir in your favorite vegetables, cooked or raw. Makes a great accompaniment to rice or quinoa.

Cheeky Chili

Serves four
20 mins
Blender, food processor

> I first made this on Christmas Day 2006. It's bright red because of the beetroot, and I served it with Macauliflower Cheese (p. 113) and Christal Kale (p. 116), so the plates were a beautiful Christmassy red, white and green.

5 tomatoes
2 red chili peppers
1 small bunch cilantro
1 cup (100 g) goji berries
2 Tbsp tamari
2 Tbsp apple cider vinegar
4 Tbsp cold-pressed, extra-virgin olive oil
4 small (250 g) beets
2 carrots
1 cup (100 g) mixed bean sprouts
¾ cup (100 g) cacao nibs

Chop the tomatoes into pieces small enough for your blender. Deseed the chili. Loosely chop the cilantro. Put the tomatoes, chili and cilantro in the blender with the gojis, tamari, vinegar, olive oil, and blend. Peel the beets, chop into quarters, and using the S-blade on your food processor, process it into small pieces about the size of rice granules. Transfer the beets to a large mixing bowl. Top and tail the carrots, quarter them, and process in the same way. Transfer to the bowl with the bean sprouts and cacao nibs and give it all a good stir together with a large spoon. Pour over the goji sauce and stir again so it is evenly mixed.

Popeye Loves You

Serves two
10 mins
No equipment needed

He also loves Olive Oil, which is why I used it in this recipe, but you can use hemp or flax oil if you prefer. Eat this for dinner and you'll be tearing up sails and lifting anchors like the man himself.

2 Tbsp cold-pressed, extra-virgin olive oil
1 Tbsp raw tahini
2 Tbsp maca
1 tsp brown unpasteurized miso
2 Tbsp nori flakes
2 cups (100 g) spinach
1 cup (100 g) sauerkraut

Make a dressing in a small bowl using the olive oil, tahini, maca and miso. Give it a good stir with a spoon until it's blended. In a larger bowl, mix the spinach, sauerkraut and nori with the dressing. Give it all a good mix. If you want to leave it, anything from a couple of hours to a couple of days, the spinach will wilt into the sauce just like it does when it's cooked.

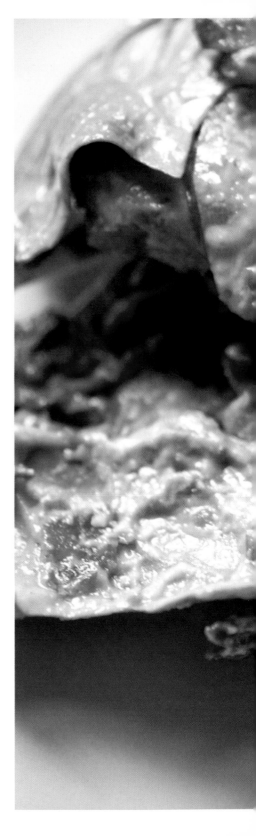

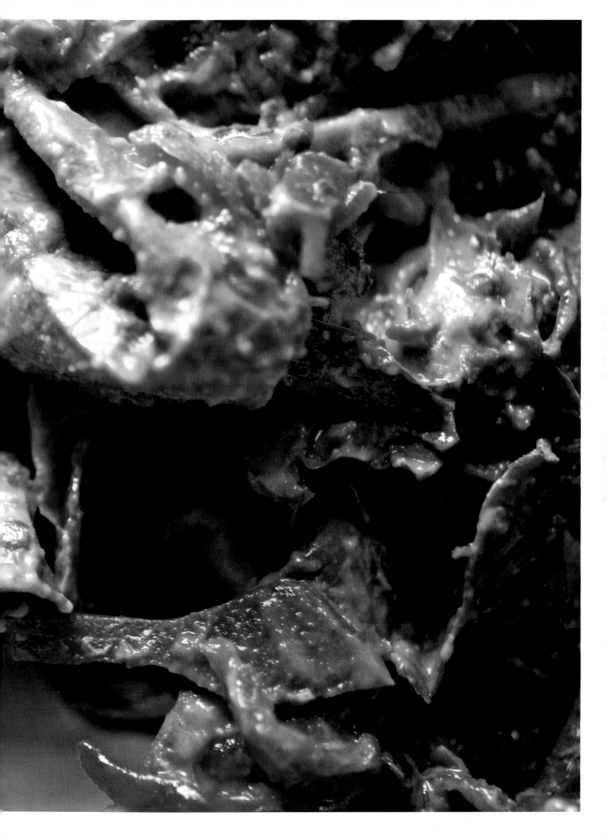

Mermaid Soup

Serves two
10 mins
Blender

> I made this for the mermaids who live off Brighton Beach. I think they would be proud. In fact, if you catch them at dusk, you'll see them dancing on the rocks.

1 ⅛ cups (250 ml) water, boiled
1 cucumber
2 stalks celery
1 avocado
4 sheets nori
2 Tbsp spirulina
½ tsp kelp
1 tsp cumin

Heat the water in your kettle. Chop the cucumber and celery into pieces to fit into your blender. Scoop the flesh out of the avocado and spoon that into the blender as well. Tear the nori sheets into quarters, and put them in along with the spirulina, kelp and cumin. Blend it all up to a cream, then pour the water in gradually as the blender is turning. Eat immediately.

Dehydrated Savories

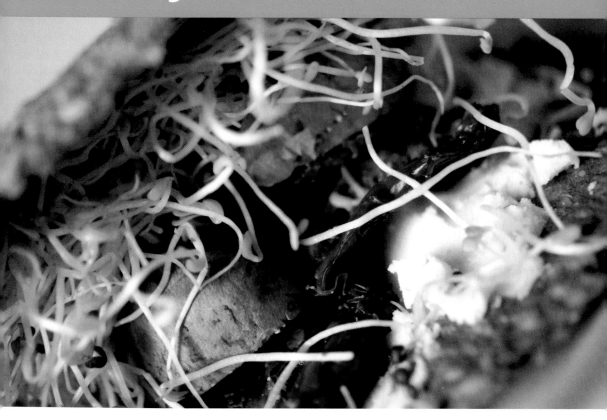

Sorry, but you need a dehydrator for all the recipes in this section. A dehydrator is like a raw-fooder's oven; it heats things at a very low temperature, so they are still technically considered raw as they are still enzymatically active, but foods get dried out enough to change them from soft doughs and batters to firm loaves and crispy crackers. If you don't have a dehydrator, you can still make most of these recipes in a fan oven, on the lowest setting, although they probably won't be raw that way.

Crackables

Makes 60 crackers
10 mins, 12 hours presoaking,
    18 hours dehydrating
Blender, dehydrator

Flax crackers are a raw food staple. They make a cool snack because they go with anything, they add that extra crunch to any dinner, and they're infinitely variable. Simply soak flaxseeds in water, add any flavoring you choose, sweet or savory, and dehydrate until crispy. Here we've put them with barleygrass to make the healthiest crackers on the block.

2 cups (250 g) flaxseeds,
    presoaked 12 hours
4 cups (1 liter) water
1 red onion
4 Tbsp barleygrass powder
2 lemons, juiced

Soak the flaxseeds in the water for 12 hours. When it's ready, put the flax and water mixture in the blender. Peel and quarter the onion and put that in too with the barleygrass powder and lemon juice. Blend until you have a puree, with no seedy bits or onion chunks left. Spread over three dehydrator trays and dry for 12 hours. Score into 20 crackers to each tray, flip, and dry for a further six hours. Store them in an airtight container and they'll keep for two to three months.

Fire Wizard Crackers

Makes 60 crackers
10 mins, 12 hours presoaking,
    18 hours dehydrating
Dehydrator

Eat these and be burning up with magical powers! If you're a big chili fan, you can slice up a red chili pepper and add that into the mix too for extra fire.

2 cups (250 g) flaxseeds,
    presoaked 12 hours
3 cups (750 ml) water
1 tsp purple corn extract
1 Tbsp Thai vegan curry powder
½ tsp crystal salt
2 lemons, juiced
1 cup (100 g) bee pollen

Soak the water in the flaxseeds overnight. When it's ready, the seeds will have absorbed all the water and be one gloopy mass. Stir in the remaining ingredients by hand, until the purple corn extract is evenly distributed in the flax and the result is an amazing purple colour. Spread over three dehydrator trays, and dry for 12 hours. Score each tray into 20 crackers, four across by five down, and flip them over to dry through on the other side. Dry for a further six hours. Store them in an airtight container, and they'll keep for up to eight weeks.

Omega Love Loaf

Serves 12
15 mins, dehydrating 12 hours
Blender, dehydrator

If you have a nut allergy, or are catering for someone who has, you can still make a "nut loaf" using flaxseeds instead. Flaxseeds are a great binder, and make a chewy, bread-like dough. You don't need to put suma in this if you don't have any, but it gives it that extra love factor.

2 cups (250 g) flaxseeds
3 (250 g) carrots
2 red onions
2 (250 g) beets
1 ½ cup (150 g) goji berries
½ cup (50 g) sun-dried tomatoes
1 Tbsp purple corn extract
1 Tbsp suma
1 Tbsp cumin powder
1 Tbsp tamari
2 Tbsp goji berries
2 Tbsp shelled hemp seeds
1 tsp purple corn extract

Grind the flaxseeds. Prepare your carrot, pepper, onion, celery and beetroot for the blender by removing unwanted seeds and stems, and chopping into pieces small enough to work your machine comfortably. You need to peel the beets. If you have a high-power blender, use this, otherwise a food processor will do fine. Put all the veg in first, with 150 g (1 ½ cups) goji berries, and the sun-dried tomatoes and blend for a few minutes until it's as broken down as it's going to get. Add the flaxseeds, purple corn extract, suma, cumin and tamari, and process again until you have a dough. Remove the dough from the mixer and shape onto a dehydrator tray, about 5 cm (1") high. I like to make it into a heart shape, but you can make whatever shape you choose. Decorate with goji berries, a sprinkling of purple corn extract and hemp seeds, radiating out in a concentric pattern. Dehydrate for at least 12 hours. Store in the fridge in an airtight container, and it will keep for up to a week.

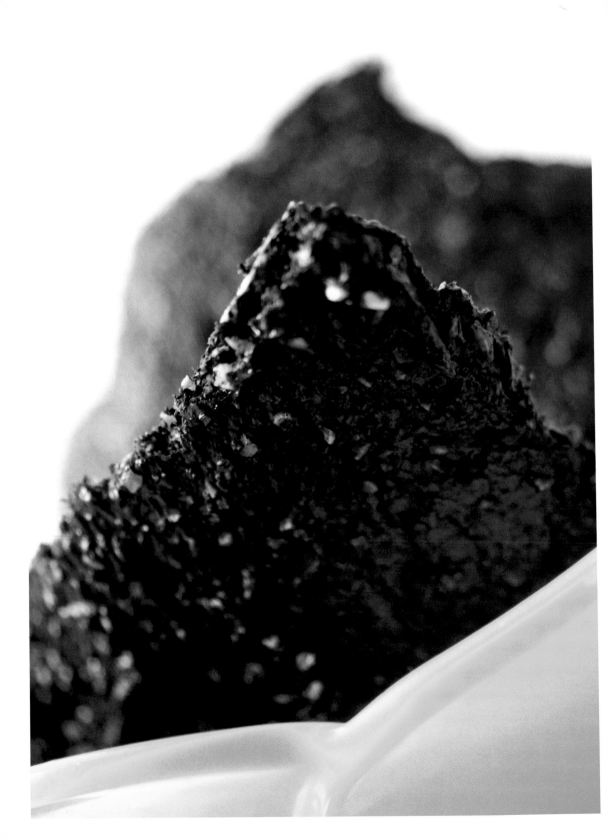

Green Goddesses

Makes 25 biscuits
15 mins, 12 hours presoaking,
   18 hours dehydrating
Blender

> These little babies go gorgeous topped with avocado and alfalfa sprouts. Lots of AmAzing foods begin with A—apples, artichokes, asparagus, angel delight….

2 cups (350 g) pumpkin seeds,
   presoaked 12 hours
½ cup (75 g) flaxseeds
2 cups (500 ml) water
1 cup (100 g) spirulina
1 Tbsp tamari
1 large red onion
1 Tbsp Seagreens or other
   sea vegetable granules

Soak the pumpkin seeds overnight or for at least four hours. When they're ready, drain them and add them to your blender with the dry flaxseed, spirulina, tamari, and water. Prepare your onion by peeling and quartering it and add that in too. Blend it all together for a couple of minutes until there are no seedy bits or onion chunks visible. Stir in the Seagreens by hand. Spread over one dehydrator tray, and dry for 12 hours. At this point, score them into biscuits, five across by five down and flip them over. Dry them for another six hours. They make quite a moist biscuit, so store in the fridge and eat within two weeks or they will start going moldy

Flaxtastic Olive Bread

Serves eight
10 mins, 18 hours dehydrating
Blender, dehydrator

> Kind of like raw ciabatta, you can add whatever you like to this gourmet bread—sun-dried tomatoes, poppy seeds, oregano, basil….

1½ cups (250 g) flaxseed, ground
1 red onion
2 tsp brown unpasteurized miso
1 cup (250 ml) water
1 cup (100 g) pitted olives
1 Tbsp Seagreens or other
   sea vegetable granules

You need to use dry flaxseed for this to get the doughy effect. Pre-grind it first in a coffee grinder, spice mill, or high-power blender. Peel your onion and cut it into at least eight pieces. Put the flax, onion, miso and water in the blender and quite quickly it should turn into a stiff dough. Stir in the olives and Seagreens by hand. Shape into a loaf about 5 cm (2") high—make it whatever shape you like, circles, hearts, and parallelograms are all good. Dehydrate for 12 hours, then flip over and dry for a further six hours on the other side. It'll still be soft and moist on the inside. Store in the fridge and eat within a week.

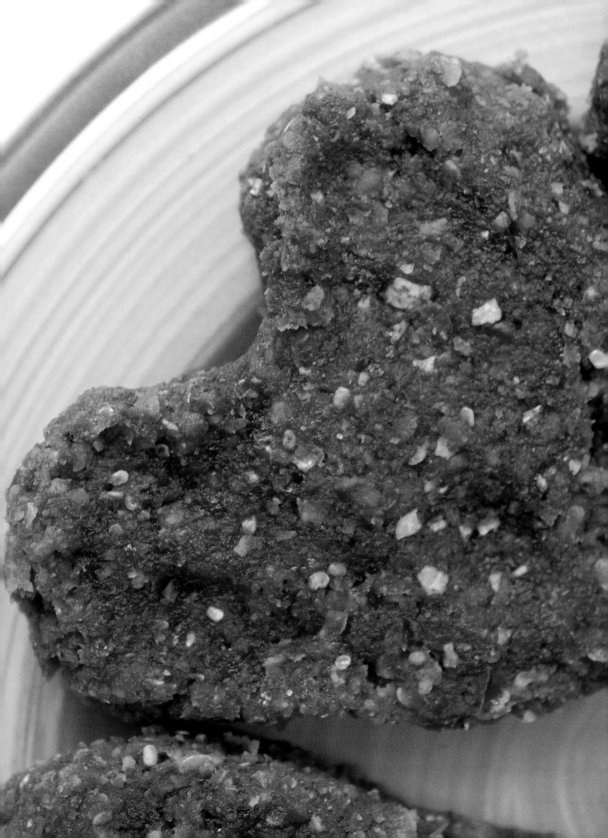

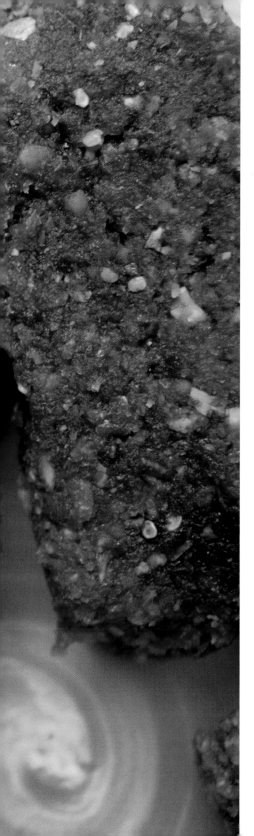

Love Burgers

Makes 12 burgers
15 mins, 12 hours presoaking,
    12 hours drying
Blender, dehydrator

> Gojis and almonds are a good combination, gojis and garlic are a good combination, gojis and carrots are a good combination. These are good.

2 cups (250 g) almonds,
    soaked 12 hours
⅓ cup (50 g) flaxseed, ground
2 tomatoes
1 carrot
Small bunch cilantro
1 cup (100 g) gojis
2 cloves garlic
1 Tbsp tamari
1 tsp Chaga or other
    mushroom extract

Presoak the almonds overnight, or for at least four hours. When they are ready, drain them. If you have a high-power blender you can make your burgers in that; if not use a food processor. Grind your flaxseeds if you haven't already done so. Chop the tomatoes, carrot and cilantro into small pieces to fit comfortably into your machine. Put everything in together and blend to a thick paste. With your hands, shape into burgers about 1 cm high and 5 cm in diameter. Dry for about nine hours, then flip over and dry for three hours more. When they're crunchy on both sides, they're done. Will keep in an airtight container in the fridge for up to a week.

Choccoli Biscuits

Makes 50 biscuits
10 mins, presoaking 12 hours, drying 18 hours
Blender, dehydrator

Choccoli = chocolate broccoli, two of our favorite foods combined. If you have purple kale or purple sprouting broccoli, you can make beautiful purple choccolis. These are gorgeous spread with some Many Ways Mayonnaise (p. 97) and heaped with alfalfa sprouts.

1 cup (125 g) brazilnuts
½ cup (75 g) flaxseeds
2 cups (500 ml) water
1 head (250 g) broccoli
1 red onion
½ cup (50 g) cacao nibs
4 Tbsp apple cider vinegar

Presoak the brazil nuts and flaxseeds together in a bowl with the water overnight. When you are ready, pour the mixture into the blender. Chop the broccoli into small pieces and add that in too. Peel and quarter the onion and pop that in with the nibs and vinegar. Blend to a thick puree so there are no bits of brazil nuts or broccoli left in. Spread evenly over two dehydrating trays. Dry for 12 hours, then score each sheet into pieces, five across by five down. Flip the biscuits over and dry for another six hours. When they're ready, transfer to an airtight container and they will keep for up to two weeks.

Burger Me

Makes 10 burgers
15 mins, 18 hours dehydrating
Blender, dehydrator

> Serve with goji ketchup (p. 94), cacaoslaw (p. 111) and camu get me (p. 248) and Mickey D's can go swivel.

1 cup (150 g) hemp seed
2 Tbsp flaxseed, ground
1 cup (150 g) cacao nibs
1 red onion
Small bunch basil
2 carrots
4 stalks celery
4 dates
1 Tbsp brown unpasteurized miso
½ tsp Reishi or other medicinal mushroom extract

Grind the hemp seeds, flaxseeds and cacao nibs first in a coffee grinder or high-power blender. Then prepare all your veg by peeling and chopping into small pieces—onions, basil, carrot, celery and dates. Break them down in a high-power blender or your food processor. Then, in whichever machine you are using, put all your ingredients—seeds, nibs, veg reishi and miso—together and mix for a few minutes until everything is amalgamated. Shape into patties about 1 cm high and 5 cm in diameter, and dry for 12 hours. Flip and dry for another six hours. Store in the fridge in an airtight container for up to a week.

Chiccolis

Serves six
15 mins, 2 hours setting
No equipment needed

> If I had to pick one genius idea out of this book, this might well be the one. Chili-flavored, chocolate-coated broccoli. Kind of on a Heston Blumenthal tip, i.e. combining unlikely ingredients into a dish that works surprisingly brilliantly. Also works with celery (chocery), red pepper, olives (chocolives), even seaweed, whatever you fancy.

1 cup (110 g) cacao butter
1 cup (90 g) cacao powder
¾ cup (75 g) mesquite powder
½ tsp chili powder
½ tsp salt
1 head (250 g) broccoli

Start to make the chocolate by melting the cacao butter (p. 78). Put the cacao powder, mesquite, chili and salt in a bowl, and mix them together with a spoon. Pour in the cacao butter and stir into a cream. Take your broccoli and snap off the individual florets, dipping them into the chocolate as thoroughly as you can. Lay them out on a large plate or tray and leave them in the fridge to set for a couple of hours. Serve as a snack or as an accompaniment to a salad for dinner.

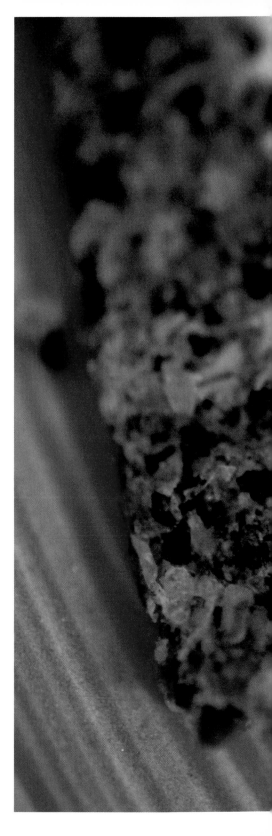

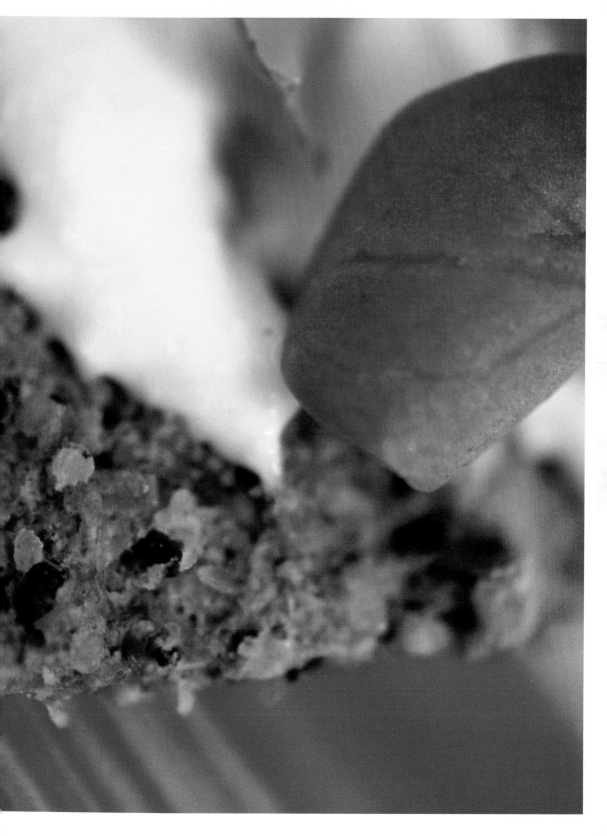

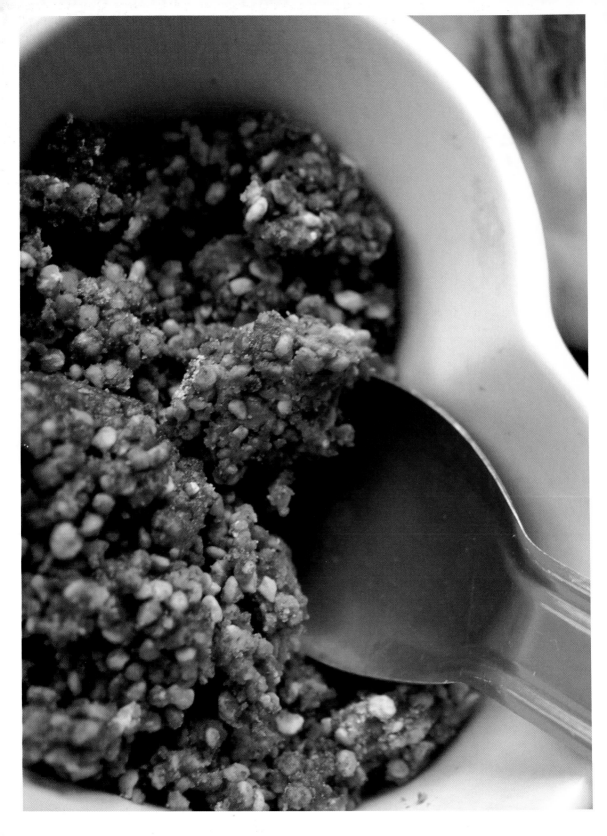

Desserts and Breakfasts

Why are desserts and breakfasts in the same section, you may be asking? Because with Raw Magic they're interchangeable! Your desserts are so healthy you can eat them for breakfast, and your breakfasts are so good you'll want them for dessert. Chocfast = chocolate for breakfast, Pudfast = pudding for breakfast, and Cakefast is for those mornings when you know you need a triumphant kickstart to your day.

Perfect Pollen

Serves two
5 mins
No equipment needed

How can I explain in words just how perfect this little combination is? It just does something to me that makes me feel that life is perfect again, that everything is just as it should be, and good things always come to those who wait. On those days when I've got too much to do and no time to think, this is my lifesaver.

1 cup (100 g) bee pollen
2 Tbsp lucuma powder
1 Tbsp raw tahini
1 Tbsp flax oil
2 Tbsp water
¼ tsp purple corn extract
½ tsp Crystal Manna
   or E3 AFA flakes
1 tsp cacao powder
1 tsp raw honey

Mix everything together in a bowl with a spoon, and try not to eat it all at once unless you want to be flying 'round the flowers in ecstasy.

Cape Town Chia

Serves four
Takes five minutes to make, but then you need to leave it soaking for at least
    a couple of hours
No equipment needed

Chia is one of my favorite foods, and this recipe is one of my favorite ways of using it. Chia is one of the very best sources of those all-important essential fatty acids, and is a superb source of energy. This pudding makes a great breakfast food, or a healthy between-meals snack. Baobab is another favorite ingredient! It is a South African superfruit with a light sweet/sour flavor that tantalizes your tastebuds and enhances every dish you care to add it to.

    4 cups (1 liter) hemp milk
    1 cup (150 g) chia seeds
    1 cup (100 g) raisins or goji berries
    2 Tbsp Baobab powder

If you haven't already done so, make your hemp milk now, by blending two tablespoons of shelled hemp into a liter of water. Hemp is my favorite, but you can try this with almond milk, or, if you prefer, milk from a carton such as rice milk or soy milk.

In a big bowl, place your chia, and then pour your milk over it. Give it a good stir with a spoon. You may find you get lumps of chia, which it's easiest to break down with a fork. Add in the raisins and baobab, and stir them in so they are evenly mixed. The sweetness of the raisins is absorbed into the pudding, so there's no need for extra sweeteners. Leave to stand for at least two hours, until the milk is fully absorbed into the chia. You may need to stir it intermittently to make sure there are no lumps.

If you don't want to eat it all straightaway, this pudding will keep well in the fridge (in fact, it improves with age) for up to five days.

Purple Power Pudding

Serves one
5 mins
Blender

Purple corn extract and cinnamon is an exceptionally tasty combination, and this pudding combines them with Etherium Black to produce a treat that makes you feel empurpled and empowered.

1 large avocado
1 Tbsp tahini
2 Tbsp lucuma powder
1 Tbsp agave nectar
½ cup (100 ml) water
1 tsp purple corn extract
⅛ tsp Etherium Black
1 tsp cinnamon

Peel and pit the avocado. Put all the ingredients in the blender together and blend for a minute until smooth. Serve topped with blueberries, blackberries, or chopped figs—any purplicious fruit.

Omegoji Pudding

Serves four
10 mins, 1 hour presoaking
Blender

Oh my gojiness! Breakfast, lunch or dinner, this pudding will have you smiling for your country, scraping out the bowl, and then dancing 'round the room in pure brain-food bliss.

1 cup (100 g) goji berries
½ cup (50 g) shelled hemp seeds
½ cup (50 g) flaxseeds
2 avocados
1 Tbsp hemp oil
1 Tbsp flax oil
2 Tbsp xylitol or coconut palm sugar
2 Tbsp agave nectar
1 cup (250 ml) water
1 Tbsp shelled hemp seeds
1 Tbsp goji berries

Soak the goji berries in advance in pure water. Once they're ready, drink the soak water—it's delicious and nutritious. Put the hemp and flax in the blender and grind up to a powder. Then add in the soaked gojis, avocados, oils, xylitol and agave nectar and blend again to a cream. Keep blending, slowly adding the water in. Once it's completely blended, transfer to two serving bowls and decorate with the remaining hemp seeds and goji berries.

Raw Magic Heaven

Serves one
5 mins
No equipment needed

My friend Alex and I invented this one day in our Raw Magic shop back in 2006. It blew our sneakers off. Since then I crave it if I'm feeling a little down or depleted. If this doesn't get you back into raw magic heaven, nothing will.

200 g Gorgeous Goji pudding (p. 167)
1 Be the Change bar (or 40 g of any raw chocolate bar)
50 g Magic Mix (or any raw trail mix)
1 Blue Manna or E3 AFA Mend capsule

Make the goji pudding from the recipe on p. 167. Cut a Be the Change bar (or 40 g of your favorite raw chocolate) into small nibble-sized pieces. Stir it into the pudding with half a bag of Magic Mix. If you haven't got Magic Mix you could just use goji berries and yacon root, or your favorite raw trail mix. Empty out the Blue Manna capsule into the pudding and stir it in. Eat and be transported into an instant whirlwind of over-excitement.

Lemon Deelite

Serves four
Time needed: 3–7 days presoaking, 10 minutes to make, 4 hours to set
Blender

> I am a confirmed Irish moss addict—nothing beats it for making light but satisfying desserts. Like kale chips and kelp noodles, Irish moss desserts are something you tuck into, feeling that they are so good they must be sinful, and then get a spark of elation when you realize you are actually eating some of the most nutrient-dense food on the planet and you can eat to your heart's content.

1 oz or 30 g Irish moss, prepared as below
4 cups (1 liter) almond milk
2 Tbsp lecithin
1 cup or 100 g lucuma powder
2 lemons (peeled)
2 Tbsp agave nectar
½ cup or 60 g coconut oil (melted)

It seems there's a bit of a knack to Irish moss. It's not the easiest of ingredients to use, but once you've made friends with it, you'll find it was well worth the effort. This is the method we have found works with the red moss that we have in Europe. If you are using the white kind, it may behave differently, so please check the manufacturer's instructions carefully to ensure the best results. If you get it wrong, your dessert will taste of seaweed, which probably isn't the end result you are after.

Take your moss and rinse it well. Then find an airtight container to house it in, and put the moss and 1 cup (250 ml) pure water in the tub. Put the lid on and leave it in the fridge. We find our moss likes a minimum of three days soaking, and up to seven days. When you're ready to use it, throw away the soak water, and make sure NOT to rinse the moss again. Blend it up with 1 cup (250 ml) of the almond milk. Blend it for a good few minutes until the moss is broken down as much as possible, and the mixture starts to go light and fluffy. At the same time you can be melting your coconut oil if necessary.

Then add the lecithin, lucuma, agave and lemon flesh and blend again, also for a few minutes, until you have a thick cream. Add the coconut oil, blend again and then gradually add the remaining 750 ml (3 cups) of almond milk. Whip it for another good minute, then pour out into a large mold or serving dish. Refrigerate for at least four hours and then serve as is or with seasonal berries.

We can't tell you how long it keeps because we've never any left long enough, but we'd guess up to a week.

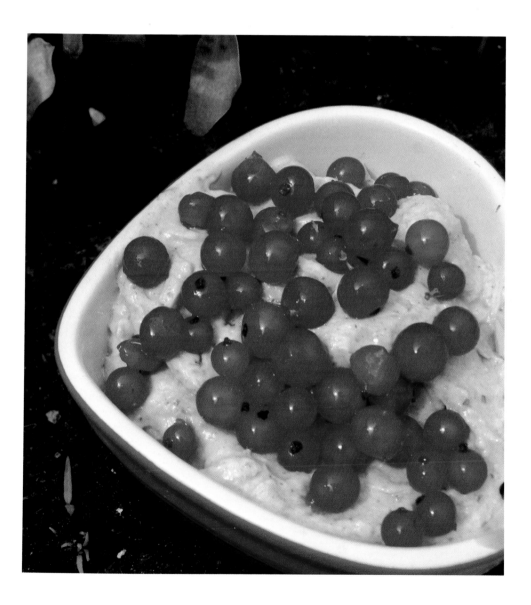

Goji Mash-Up

Serves two
5 mins
No equipment needed

We invented this on a long drive one day when we didn't have access to a blender. We wanted dessert so we just threw together what we had and hey presto! As if by magic, a new favorite was born. Like goji pudding but without the hassle of actually making it.

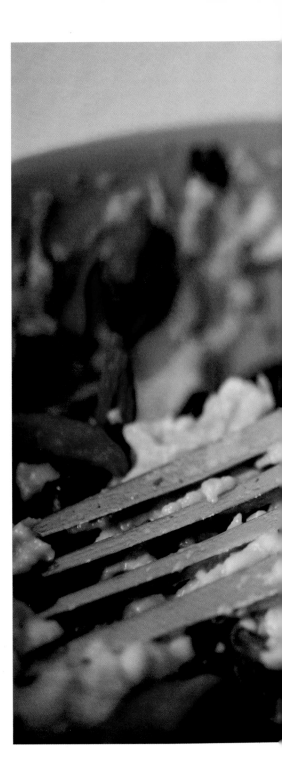

2 avocados
2 tsp agave nectar
2 Tbsp raw tahini
4 Tbsp goji berries
2 Tbsp cacao nibs

Scoop the avocado flesh out into a bowl with a spoon. Using a fork, mash it up as much as possible. Add the remaining ingredients into the bowl and mash again, making sure the agave nectar and tahini are evenly mixed in. Eat, and then get back in the car with some very good music to play loudly as you zoom down the freeway.

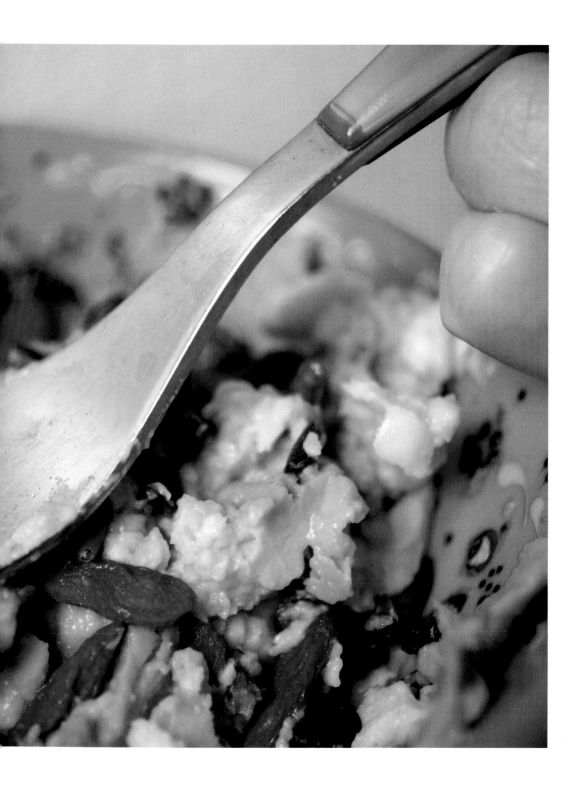

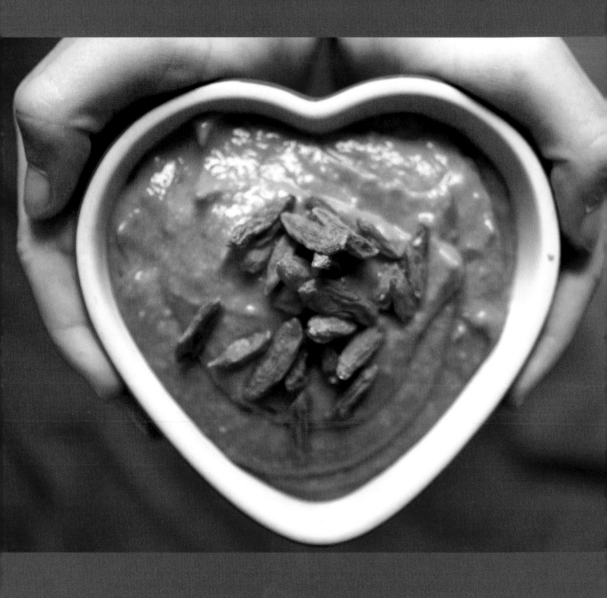

Gorgeous Goji Pudding

Serves two
10 mins, 1 hour presoaking
Blender

This was our best seller in the Raw Magic shop, after the chocolate. It's indulgent but also really refreshing and invigorating. The boys have it for breakfast as a treat. Seven years after first inventing it, it's still one of my all-time favorite desserts.

1 cup (100 g) goji berries, soaked 1 hour
2 avocados
2 Tbsp coconut oil
2 Tbsp agave nectar
2 Tbsp lucuma powder
1 Tbsp camu
½ lemon, juiced
2 cups (500 ml) water
additional 1 Tbsp goji berries

Soak the gojis in pure water one hour in advance. Drain, and drink the soak water, it's delicious. Remove the flesh from the avocados and put it in the blender. Add the coconut oil (you don't have to melt it first, it will break down in the blender), agave nectar, lucuma, camu, lemon juice and water. Give it all a whiz, then add the water slowly, keeping the blender running. When you have a thick dollopy pudding, it's ready to serve. Sprinkle with gojis to decorate. Or try crumbling a chocolate bar into it—have a look at Raw Magic Heaven on p. 161.

Call the Police

Serves two
10 mins
Blender

I've made some of my best food when I've been heartbroken. As my friend Shazzie once said, "Chocolate or men? At least you get an answer out of chocolate." There's no better way of reaffirming your status as a beautiful being when you've been rejected by a guy who doesn't know a good thing when he sees it, than getting in the kitchen and creating yourself some gorgeousness. I called this Call the Police because it's so good it should be illegal. A bit like me.

½ cup (50 g) cacao butter
2 avocados
1 Tbsp agave nectar
1 cup (100 g) mesquite powder
½ cup (50 g) cacao powder
½ tsp suma
1 ½ cups (375 ml) water
1 Tbsp cacao nibs
1 Tbsp goji berries

To start, melt the cacao butter. Remove the flesh from the avocados and put it in the blender with the agave nectar, mesquite, cacao powder, suma and melted butter. Blend it all up and then add the water gradually, keeping the blender turning. Serve decorated with cacao nibs and goji berries.

Green Gloop

Serves four
10 mins
Blender

This recipe reminds me of the glorious Gela of rawreform.com. When we lived together, we both had this affliction called Spirulina Mouth, which involved eating large quantities of spirulina, then smiling at someone and scaring them with our deep green teeth and lips. For some reason, delivery men love to ring on the door just when you're eating spirulina.

2 avocados
1 cup (100 g) lucuma powder
½ cup (50 g) spirulina
3 Tbsp agave nectar
1 cup (250 ml) water

Scoop the flesh out of the avocados and put it in the blender with the lucuma, spirulina, agave nectar and half the water. Put the blender on and slowly add the rest of the water until you have quite a thick pudding. Keeps in the fridge for up to a week. If you just can't help yourself, you can add 50 g (½ cup) chocolate powder and some extra agave nectar to taste, and turn this into a secretly chocolatey green gloop.

Goji Porridge

Serves four
10 mins, 12 hours presoaking
Blender

Most oats sold commercially in the UK are steamed to stabilize them or they go rancid. At Raw Living, we have sourced fresh raw oats that are packed specially for us. They only have a shelf life of eight weeks, but the difference in flavor is amazing. If you are into your raw foods, it is worth getting hold of some. If you're using heat-treated oats, they are still a good source of fuel, and balancing for the blood sugar.

2 cups (250 g) rolled oats, soaked overnight
½ cup (50 g) goji berries, soaked 1 hour
2 Tbsp xylitol
2 cups (500 ml) water
Additional 2 Tbsp goji berries
2 Tbsp raisins

Soak the oats overnight. Soak the goji berries an hour in advance. Drink the soak water when they're ready, it's wondrous. Drain the oats and put them in the blender with the gojis, xylitol and water. Blend it up, it will seem really runny, but it will thicken once heated. Put in a large pan and heat very gently over a low heat, keeping it under 118° F if possible (this is the temperature at which enzymes are destroyed and food stops technically being raw). Stir in the raisins and gojis. After about five minutes of stirring it should thicken nicely. Serve immediately. If you don't want to eat it all at once, the mixture will keep in the fridge for up to a week and you can just heat up as much as you need at a time.

Maca Porridge

Serves four
10 mins, presoaking 12 hours
Blender

Oats and maca are a really good combination. Both are stabilizing to the blood sugar, and give a long-lasting energy boost. Have this for breakfast and you'll feel calm, strong and capable of taking on anything the universe throws at you! If you're just making it for yourself, you can blend up a batch and keep it in the fridge, heating up just what you need each day.

2 cups (250 g) rolled oats, soaked overnight
4 Tbsp maca
4 Tbsp lucuma powder
2 Tbsp xylitol or coconut palm sugar
1 Tbsp cinnamon
2 cups (500 ml) water
2 Tbsp goji berries
2 Tbsp raisins

Soak the oats overnight in pure water. In the morning drain them and put in the blender with the maca, lucuma, xylitol, cinnamon and water. Blend it all up to a milk; it will be very runny still. Put in the pan and heat very gently over a low heat for five minutes. A porringer or double saucepan is ideal for this. Keep it under 118° F if you can, which is the temperature at which enzymes are killed and it stops being "officially" raw. Stir in the raisins and gojis. Eat immediately while warm.

Purple Mayhem

Serves two
5 mins
No equipment needed

Breakfast madness. If you want to start your day in a tripped-out purple haze, try this for size. Or you could end your day this way too. Or if you want real mayhem, have it at both ends of the day.

    1 Tbsp cacao powder
    1 tsp purple corn extract
    2 Tbsp mesquite powder
    1 Tbsp raw tahini
    1 Tbsp agave nectar
    2 Tbsp water
    1 cup (100 g) buckwheaties (see p. 78)

Put the cacao powder, purple corn extract and mesquite in a small bowl. Pour in the tahini, agave nectar and water, and give it a good mix-up. Stir in the buckwheaties and mix again. Eat straightaway; the buckwheat will go soft if you try and keep it more than a day or two.

Orange Porridge

Serves two
10 mins
No equipment needed

This golden orange porridge is easy and fun, and a great way to ensure a sunny start to your day.

1 cup (250 ml) water, just boiled
¾ cup (100 g) flaxseeds, ground
2 Tbsp bee pollen
1 Tbsp agave nectar
2 Tbsp lucuma powder
1 Tbsp flax oil

Boil the water. Grind the flaxseeds if you haven't already. Mix the flaxseeds, pollen, lucuma, agave nectar and flax oil together in a bowl. Gradually add the boiling water, stirring as you go, until you reach the desired consistency. Eat it straightaway, while it's still warm. You can make purple porridge by adding half a teaspoon of purple corn extract, or chocolate porridge with 1 Tbsp chocolate powder and a dash of extra agave nectar.

Best Ever Breakfast Cereal

Serves eight
10 mins
Dehydrator

My boys have been enjoying this for breakfast for years. Sprouted buckwheat is a wonderful food, really grounding and calming but still light. Buckwheat is technically a seed, not a grain, and it's superbly alkalizing. You can vary it with any berry you like—try substituting mulberries for cranberries, or cacao nibs for bee pollen.

2 cups (200 g) buckwheaties (see p. 78)
1 cup (100 g) goji berries
1 cup (100 g) bee pollen
1 cup (100 g) dried cranberries
¾ cup (100 g) shelled hemp seeds
2 Tbsp raw tahini
2 Tbsp flax oil
2 Tbsp agave nectar
4 Tbsp lucuma powder
1 tsp crystal salt
1 Tbsp probiotics powder

In a large mixing bowl, put the buckwheat, gojis, pollen, cranberries, and hemp. Give it all a good mix together. In a small separate bowl, pour the tahini, flax oil, agave nectar, lucuma, salt and probiotics. Stir it all up to a thick paste with a small spoon. Pour it over the buckwheat mix, and give it a really good mix, making sure it's evenly coating it. Store in an airtight container; it will keep in the fridge for up to a week. Don't add water to the mix or this will make the buckwheat go soggy.

Chocolate Chipper Nicest Icest Cream

Serves four
5 mins, 20 mins freezing
Blender, ice cream maker

Who doesn't love chocolate ice cream? For a double chocolate treat, crumble a raw chocolate bar into the ice cream.

2 cups (250 g) shelled hemp seeds
¾ cup (75 g) cacao powder
⅓ cup (60 g) xylitol or
    coconut palm sugar
1 cup (100 g) mesquite powder
1 ½ cups (375 ml) water
1 cup (100 g) cacao nibs

Blend up everything apart from the nibs. These are your choc-chips, stir them in afterwards, once everything's blended to a cream. Pour into the ice cream maker, and proceed according to the manufacturer's instructions. If you don't have an ice cream maker, you can pour it into a Tupperware tub or Pyrex bowl, and leave it in the freezer for a couple of hours until it's soft and scoopable.

Hempilicious Ice Cream

Serves four
5 mins, 20 mins freezing
Blender, ice cream maker

Ice cream makers are the best and easiest way I know of making raw ice cream, and hopefully you will have realized by now that raw ice cream is a pretty essential part of life. If you don't have one, you can just put the mix in the freezer for a couple of hours until it's frozen enough for you.

2 cups (250 g) shelled hemp seeds
1 cups (100 g) lucuma powder
⅓ cup (45 g) xylitol
    or coconut sugar
1 Tbsp purple corn extract
1 ½ cups (375 ml) water

Put everything in the blender and blend to a cream. Pour into your ice cream maker and blend according to the manufacturer's instructions. Eat served with strawberries and goji berries on a hot summer's day for some hempilicious heavenliness.

Cakes and Cookies

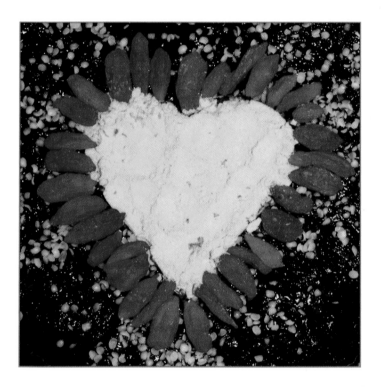

Have I mentioned that finally, for the first time in human history, we truly can have our cake and eat it? That the world has never seen cakes the likes of these before? So sublimely, divinely, orgasmically, beautifully inspired, they defy description? So bursting with love on all levels, physical, emotional, mental and spiritual, that you will wonder how it has taken us so many millennia to get to this pinnacle of human existence. Well, you will wonder for a minute, then you will take another bite of cake and not worry about anything much anymore other than the next seed of bliss you can plant, the next gift of love you can give.

Best Ever Brownies

Makes 25
10 mins, 8–12 hours presoaking, 18 hours drying
Blender, dehydrator

These are based around the flapjack recipe from my first book, *Eat Smart, Eat Raw*. There are a lot of recipes in that book that I still use on a daily basis, and the flapjacks are one of them, but they have to be the ace in the pack. They taste so good, you'll be saying, "I can't believe they're not baked."

2 cups (250 g) oats, soaked 8–12 hours
1 ½ cups (175 g) cacao nibs
4 Tbsp agave nectar
¼ cup (60 ml) water
½ cup (125 ml) cold-pressed, extra-virgin olive oil
1 Tbsp maca powder
2 Tbsp mesquite powder
½ cup (60 g) mulberries (raisins will do if you can't find them)

Soak the oats overnight. When they're ready, grind up 125 g (1 cup) cacao nibs. Put all the ingredients apart from remaining 50 g (½ cup) nibs and the mulberries in the blender, and process to a thick puree. Stir in the cacao nibs and mulberries by hand. Spoon the mixture onto a dehydrating tray, about 1 cm or ½" thick. Form into a square shape. Dry for 12 hours, then score into 25 pieces (five across by five down). Turn, and dry for a further six hours. Store in an airtight container in the fridge, and eat within a couple of weeks.

Goji Bucaroonies

Makes 16
10 mins, 3 days sprouting, 18 hours dehydrating
Blender, dehydrator

Sprouted buckwheat is one of the best bases for making raw cookies. Either sprout it and dehydrate it and grind it into flour, as in the shortbread recipe (p. 180), or sprout it and blend it up for a moister cookie.

2 cups (250 g) buckwheat, sprouted 2–3 days
½ cup (60 ml) cold-pressed, extra-virgin olive oil
½ cup (60 ml) agave nectar
1 cup (100 g) gojis

Sprout the buckwheat in advance. When it's ready, blend up the buckwheat with the olive oil and agave nectar to a cream. Add the gojis to the mix and semi-blend them, so you still have bits of goji left discernible in the mix. Spread onto a dehydrator sheet and dry for 12 hours. Score into 16 cookies, four rows of four, then flip over and dehydrate for a further six hours. Will keep in an airtight container for a few weeks.

Flaxjacks

Makes 12
5 mins, 12 hours dehydrating
Blender, dehydrator

These are so easy and so satisfying. Really good coated in raw chocolate too.

1 ¼ cups (150 g) flaxseeds
1 ¼ cups (150 g) shelled hemp
seeds
3 Tbsp agave nectar
3 Tbsp water

Grind the flax and hemp to a powder using your grinder or high-power blender. Then if you've got a high-power blender, add the agave nectar and water in and blend again, otherwise transfer to a normal food processor and mix everything in there. The result should be a sticky mass. Press onto a dehydrating tray, about 1 cm (½") thick. Dry for six hours, then score into three rows by four columns. Flip over and dry for six hours more. Will keep for up to a week in an airtight container.

Whooshjaks

Makes 20 biscuits
12 hours presoaking, 10 mins,
   18 hours drying
Blender, dehydrator

Whoosh is my favorite of our raw chocolate bars. The alchemical combination of cacao, maca and suma puts me right back where I want to be every time. Blissed but energized. Add oats into the mix too and you have a truly uplifting and nourishing treat.

2 cups (250 g) oats,
   presoaked 12 hours
1 cup (100 g) cacao powder
¾ cup (75 g) maca
1 Tbsp suma
⅔ cup (100 g) xylitol
   or coconut palm sugar
½ cup (60 ml) cold-pressed,
   extra-virgin olive oil
1 cup (250 ml) water
1 cup coconut flakes

Soak the oats overnight. Drain, and add to the blender with all the remaining ingredients apart from the coconut chips. Blend for a minute or two until it's pureed. Stir in the coconut flakes, and spread on a dehydrator tray so it's about 1 cm (½") high. Dry for 12 hours, then score into biscuits four across by five down. Flip and dry for another six hours until firm. Will keep in an airtight tin for up to a week.

Macajackas

Makes 20 biscuits
12 hours presoaking, 10 mins,
 18 hours drying
Blender, dehydrator

I love maca and oats together; they really complement each other. Calming and nourishing, you feel like you can conquer the world, but actually you don't need to because everything's perfect.

2 cups (250 g) oats, presoaked
 12 hours
½ cup (50 g) maca
½ cup (50 g) mesquite powder
2 Tbsp agave nectar
2 Tbsp cold-pressed, extra-virgin
 olive oil
1 cup (100 g) raisins

Soak the oats overnight. Drain, and put in the blender with all the other ingredients apart from the raisins. Blend to a puree, then stir in the raisins by hand. Spoon out onto a dehydrator tray and spread into a square about 1 cm (½") high. Dry for 12 hours, then score into 20 biscuits, five across by four down. Dry for another six hours. Will keep in an airtight container for up to a week.

Gojackajackas

Makes 20 biscuits
12 hours presoaking, 10 mins,
 18 hours drying
Blender, dehydrator

OK, sometimes I get bored of giving you reasons to eat something. So give me one good reason not to eat these. Just one. See, you can't, can you? Nuff said.

2 cups (250 g) oats, presoaked
 12 hours
2 cups (200 g) goji berries
½ cup (50 g) lucuma powder
2 Tbsp cold-pressed, extra-virgin
 olive oil
2 Tbsp agave nectar
½ cup (60 ml) water

Presoak the oats overnight. Drain them, and add them to the blender with all the ingredients apart from 100 g gojis. Blend to a puree, then stir in the remaining gojis. Spoon onto a dehydrator tray, and shape into a rectangle, about 1 cm (½") high. Dry for 12 hours, then score into 20 biscuits, five across by four down, and flip and dry for another six hours. Stored in an airtight container, they will keep for up to two weeks.

Tarts for the Tart

Makes 12
30 mins, 2 hours setting
Blender

One week I made these and couldn't stop eating them all week; they were all I wanted. Then I went 'round to Rochelle's house and she had made almost the exact same thing. Except I didn't have a name for mine, and she did, so here it is, the Tart's Tarts. They are great to take with you when you're traveling, they'll keep you going for days. If you're a maca fan, you can substitute 50 g of the lucuma for maca. The result won't be as sweet, but it will be more energizing.

Shortbread
1 ½ cups (175 g) coconut oil
2 cups (200 g) buckwheaties
2 cups (200 g) lucuma powder
⅔ cup (100 g) xylitol or coconut sugar
1 Tbsp mucuna
1 cup (250 ml) water

Chocolate Topping
1 cup (100 g) cacao butter
½ cup (50 g) cacao powder
¾ cup (75 g) mesquite powder

Melt the coconut oil first. Grind the buckwheaties into flour in your blender. Transfer to a mixing bowl and add the lucuma, xylitol and mucuna. Give it a good mix with your hands, then pour in the melted butter and stir it in with a spoon. Add the water and stir that in too. Press into a medium-sized rectangular tin. Leave it out on the side while you make the chocolate layer.

To make the chocolate, first melt the cacao butter. Once it's liquid, remove from the heat and stir in the cacao and mesquite. Pour over the shortbread and pop it in the fridge for a couple of hours to set. Once it's hard, slice into 12 fingers, three across by four down. Will keep stored in the fridge for up to a week.

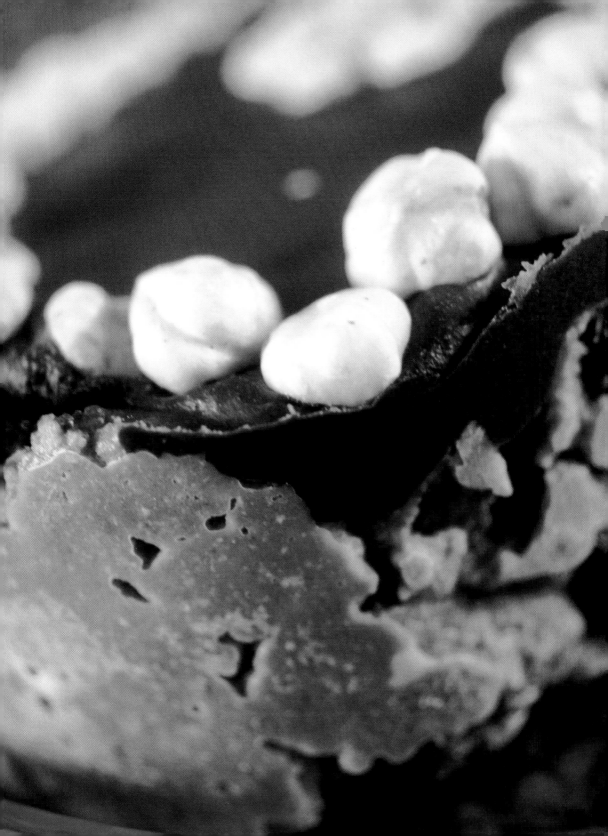

Chocolate Crispy Cakes

Makes 30 cakes
15 mins, 2 hours setting
No equipment needed

If anything in this book is too good to be true, this is it. Buy some little paper cupcake cases to put them in, and when they're ready sit down in front of a You-Tube video of your favorite kids' TV program to be transported into childhood nostalgic bliss. Then eat another one, and decide that being seven years old was pretty good, but actually here and now is the best it's ever been.

1 ¾ cups (220 g) cacao butter
2 cups (200 g) mesquite powder
1 ½ cups (150 g) cacao powder
⅓ cup (45 g) xylitol or coconut sugar
3 cups (300 g) buckwheaties (p 80)
1 ½ cups (150 g) raisins
1 ¼ cups (150 g) shelled hemp seeds

Start by melting the cacao butter. Put the mesquite, cacao powder and xylitol in a bowl, and stir in the melted butter. Quickly, stir in the buckwheaties, raisins and hemp seeds. The mixture starts to set fast, so you have to be speedy, or get someone lovely to help you so you can do it in half the time. Take large spoons of the mixture and shape into balls with your hands, about 40 g in weight, or the size of a plum. Put them in little paper muffin cups if you want, or just lay them on a tray. If you find the mixture's setting faster than you can make them into balls, you can transfer it back into your melting device and remelt a little. Put them in the fridge to set, and an hour or two later they're ready. They keep for at least four weeks in the fridge.

Kate's Cinnamon Chocolate Bread

Serves six
5 mins, dehydrating 12 hours
Blender, dehydrator

This is really filling, and so good if you split it in half through the middle and spread it with yacon syrup and pumpkin seed butter and eat it as a sandwich.

1 ¾ cups (200 g) flaxseeds
⅔ cup (100 g) cacao nibs
3 Tbsp agave nectar
1 cup (250 ml) water
1 tsp cinnamon

Grind up the cacao nibs and flaxseeds; you can do this together if you have a high-power blender, or separately in a coffee grinder. Add the remaining ingredients and blend again—the result will be a very thick sticky mass. Spoon out and press onto a dehydrator tray about 2 cm (1" high) into a loaf shape. Dehydrate for nine hours then flip over and dry on the other side for another three hours. Stored in an airtight container, it will keep for a couple of weeks.

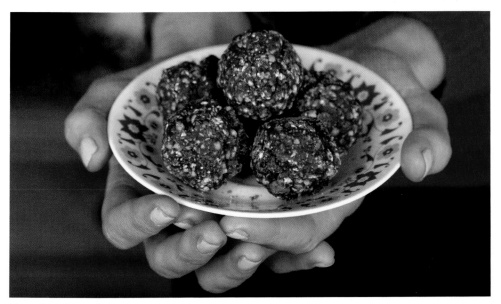

Chocolate Crispy Cakes

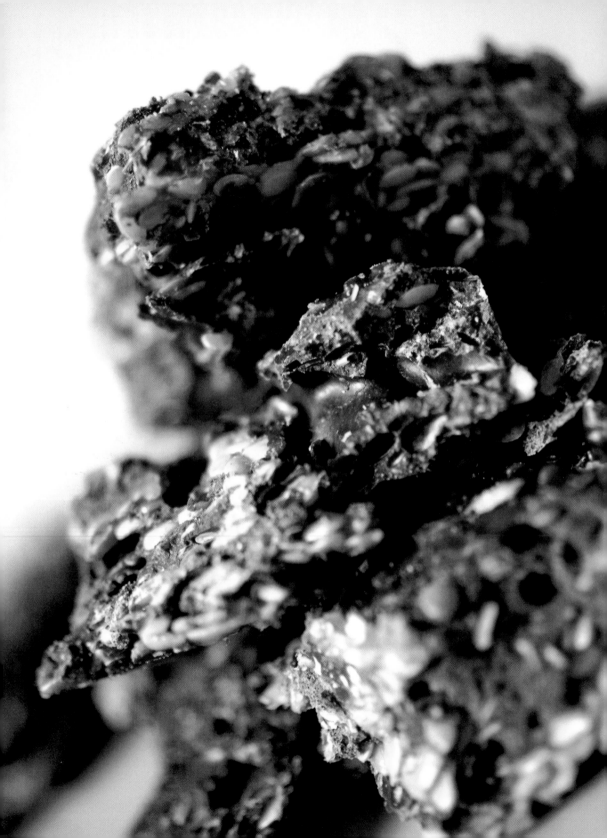

Cor It's Cornflakes Cake

Serves eight
10 mins, 12 hours presoaking, 12 hours drying, 3 hours setting
Dehydrator

This is the lazy mum's chocolate crispy cake. For those who couldn't be bothered with paper cases, we used to get this version instead, pressed flat into a tin and cut into slices.

1 ½ cups (250 g) flaxseed, presoaked 12 hours
3 cups (750 ml) pure water
1 ½ cups (180 g) cacao butter
1 ½ cups (150 g) cacao powder
1 ½ cups (150 g) mesquite powder
⅓ cup (50 g) xylitol or coconut sugar

Soak the flaxseed in the water overnight. It will swell and absorb it all. When it's ready, spread it over two dehydrator sheets and dry for about nine hours. Flip the sheets over, and dry them for another three hours, until they are fully crispy on both sides. When they're ready, it's time to make the chocolate. Melt the cacao butter first. In a bowl, mix together the cacao powder, mesquite, and xylitol. Pour in the butter and stir it all together. Take your sheets of cracker and crumble them into the chocolate, breaking them into small pieces the size of cornflakes. Give it all a good mix so the chocolate is evenly coating the crackers. Press into a Victoria sandwich tin, and leave in the fridge to set for three hours. When it's done, cut into slices, eat, and feel like you're ten years old all over again.

Gratitude Bread

Serves 10
10 mins, 12 hours drying
Grinder, dehydrator

Gratitude is one of the most powerful emotions we can express, and severely underrated in our culture where too much is never enough, and we are conditioned to always look at what we can get out of a situation rather than what we can give. Take a moment in your day to eat some bread and count your blessings, and magically the more time you find in your life to be grateful, the more you find in your life to be grateful for.

2 cups (250 g) flaxseeds
1 cup (100 g) lucuma powder
3 Tbsp agave nectar
1 Tbsp purple corn extract
½ cup (50 g) goji berries
¾ cup (200 ml) water

Grind the flaxseeds in a coffee grinder or high-power blender. Transfer them to a large mixing bowl, along with the lucuma, agave nectar, and purple corn extract, and give it all a good stir together with your hands. Add in the goji berries and mix those in too. Add the water gradually, kneading as you go, so you end up with a big stiff ball of dough. Press this onto your dehydrator tray and flatten into a loaf shape about 2 cm (1") high. Dry for nine hours, then flip and dry for a further three hours on the other side. Serve sliced through the middle and spread with any of the spreads on pages 216–219.

Surrender to the Confusion

Serves 10
10 mins, 12 hours drying
Grinder, dehydrator

Sometimes life is just too hectic and confusing and impossible to make sense of. At times like these, you need to make some of this bread, eat it, and feel that actually confusion can be quite helpful in making you surrender and let go and just relax and enjoy life a bit more.

1 ¾ cups (225 g) flaxseeds
1 cup (100 g) mesquite powder
½ cup (50 g) maca
3 Tbsp agave nectar
1 cup (100 g) dried cranberries
½ cup (150 ml) water

Grind your flaxseeds in a high-power blender or coffee grinder. Transfer them to a mixing bowl with the mesquite, maca, agave nectar, and cranberries, and give it a good mix with your hands. Then pour in the water gradually, kneading it to a dough as you go. The result should be a ball which is fairly firm, but pliable enough to shape into a loaf. Take a dehydrator tray and press your dough into a loaf shape (we like to make hearts), about 2 cm (1") high. Dry for six hours, then flip it over and dry for another six hours on the other side. Eat with any of the spreads on pages 216–219.

Bee Beautiful Bread

Serves 16
10 mins, 12 hours dehydrating
Grinder, dehydrator

If you want to be wise and wonderful, this is the stuff to have, slathered in Love Butter (p. 218). Makes a bright and beautiful breakfast.

2 ⅓ cups (300 g) flaxseeds
1 ½ cups (150 g) lucuma powder
½ cup (100 g) honey
1 cup (100 g) bee pollen
½ cup (50 g) cacao nibs
1 cup (100 g) goji berries
1 ¼ cups (300 ml) water

Grind the flaxseeds in a grinder or high-power blender. Transfer them to a mixing bowl with the lucuma, pollen, cacao and gojis, and mix it together with your hands. Pour in the honey and add the water gradually, kneading it into a ball as you go. Once you have a happy dough, shape into a loaf about 2 cm (1") high and place on a dehydrator tray. Dry for six hours, then flip over and dry for another six hours on the other side. Keeps for a couple of weeks in an airtight container.

Buzz Cake

Serves 16
15 mins, 2 hours setting
Blender

Iranian dried mulberries are becoming more popular and easy to find all the time. Try tracking them down at your local Eastern grocer or whole-food store. They're a very sweet, succulent berry that tastes like chewy honey. They go really well with pollen.

1 ⅔ cups (200 g) coconut oil
1 cup (100 g) raisins
1 cup (100 g) mulberries
1 cup (100 g) pumpkin seeds
1 cup (100 g) sunflower seeds
1 ⅔ cups (200 g) cacao nibs
1 Tbsp purple corn extract
1 cup (100 g) pollen

Melt the butter first. If you have a high-power blender, you can put everything apart from the pollen in the blender together with the coconut oil and blend to a thick cream. If you don't have a high-power blender, grind the nibs, seeds, and dried fruit separately. Then add them to the blender with the purple corn extract and coconut oil. Once it's all thoroughly mixed, stir in the pollen by hand. Press into a cake tin or flan tin and leave to set in the fridge for 2–3 hours. Cut into pieces: either 16 as a substantial pudding, or 32 for lots of little snacks. You can ice it with any of the creams and spreads on pages 216–219 if you want to make it a bit more fancy.

It Just Gets Better Biscuits

Makes 50
10 mins, 12 hours presoaking,
    12 hours dehydrating, 4 hours drying
Dehydrator

These are a bit of a faff to make, but so worth the effort. They look outstanding, with the purple cracker, red gojis, brown chocolate, white hemp and yellow pollen all complementing each other. They taste outrageously good, and they're a fantastic way to have a balanced chocolate snack, with the flaxseeds giving them more density and bite, and all that algae and extra superfoods to get you really going.

2 cups (250 g) flaxseeds,
    presoaked 12 hours
3 cups (750 ml) water
1 Tbsp purple corn extract
1 cup (100 g) goji berries,
    presoaked 1 hour

¾ cup (75 g) cacao powder
1 cup (125 g) cacao butter
1 cup (100 g) mesquite powder
1 Tbsp Crystal Manna or
    E3 AFA flakes

2 Tbsp shelled hemp seeds
2 Tbsp bee pollen

Soak the flaxseeds in the water in a large bowl overnight, or for at least four hours, until the seeds have swelled and absorbed all the water. Soak the goji berries one hour in advance. With a spoon, stir the gojis and purple corn extract into the flax batter. Give it a really good stir until the purple corn extract is evenly mixed in and it has a beautiful purple hue. Spread over two and a half dehydrator trays—not too thin, or they will break when you take them out. About two-thirds of the way through drying, remove them and score each tray into crackers, four by five. Flip them over, and let them dry through on the other side.

When they're ready, the next step is to make the chocolate. Melt the cacao butter, and when it's liquid, remove the bowl from the pan and stir in the cacao powder, mesquite and Crystal Manna. If you've got time, leave it to one side just for half an hour, so it starts to thicken very slightly, this will make it easier to stick on the biscuits. Don't leave it too long or it will set too much. Dip the end of each cracker in the chocolate, so that they are one-third to one-half covered. Mix the hemp and pollen in a bowl, and take a teaspoon at a time and sprinkle them onto one side of the chocolate, quickly before the chocolate sets. They'll look like a Zoom lolly! Lay them out on the dehydrator trays, being careful to keep them separate so they don't stick to one another (although they are pretty nice sandwiched together too), pollen side up. Unless you've got a lot of space, the best place to leave them to dry is probably in the dehydrator (don't turn it on!). They'll take about four hours to dry. When they're done store in an airtight container, they'll keep for a few weeks.

The Magic 23 Cake

Serves 12
45 mins, 1 hour presoaking, 3 hours setting
Blender

Cacao and gojis are astoundingly good together. 23 is the cosmic trigger number: when you're tuned in to the cosmic flow, when you're in the synchronicitous groove, you start seeing 23s all over the place. If you're not already in the Magic 23 place, this cake will put you there.

Filling
¾ cup (100 g) cacao butter
¾ cup (100 g) cacao nibs
1 ½ cups (150 g) goji berries, soaked 1 hour
2 (500 g) avocados
2 tsp purple corn extract
1 cup (250 ml) water
3 Tbsp agave nectar

Crust
1¼ cups (125 g) pecans
1¼ cups (125 g) oats
1¼ cups (125 g) lucuma powder
½ cup (125 ml) water

Presoak the gojis in pure water for an hour. You must drink the soak water, or use it in the cake; don't throw it away, it's divine!

To make the crust, grind up the pecans in a high-power blender or coffee grinder. Transfer them to a mixing bowl, and grind up the oats. Add them to the bowl along with the lucuma and toss it all together with your hands as if you were making normal pastry dough. Take the water, and pour it in gradually, kneading into a dough as you do so. When you have added just enough water to make it stick together in a ball, press it out into a large flan tin, lining the bottom and the sides with a crust about ½ cm thick. If you have any dough left over, you can make it into little dough balls and eat it as it is, or make it into cookies and put it in the dehydrator.

To make the filling, melt the cacao butter first. Grind the nibs in a high-power blender or coffee grinder. Drain the gojis, and put them in the blender. Scoop the flesh out of the avocados and put that in the blender too. Add in the nibs, butter, purple corn extract and agave nectar, and blend to a cream. Add the water gradually, as the blender is turning. After a minute, once you have a gorgeous smooth cream, spoon it out into your pastry case. Put in the fridge for three hours to set. Keep stored in the fridge, it will keep for up to a week.

Right Royal Tart

Serves ten
1 hour, 2 hours setting
Blender

Purple and gold together is a combination fit for royalty, to make you feel like the king or queen you really are. Eat this and reign supreme. Or better still, invite the Queen 'round for tea and offer her a slice.

Crust
1 ¼ cups (125 g) lucuma powder
1 ¼ cups (125 g) rolled oats
1 ¼ cups (125 g) almonds
1 Tbsp cinnamon
½ cup (125 ml) water

Filling
3 (750 g) avocados
1 cup (125 g) coconut oil
1 cup (100 g) mesquite powder
1 Tbsp purple corn extract
2 tsp Etherium Gold
2 Tbsp agave nectar
½ cup (125 ml) water

To make the crust, grind the almonds and oats together in a high-power blender or coffee grinder until they become flour. Transfer them to a mixing bowl and add the lucuma and cinnamon. Rub it all together with your hands, like you're making usual pastry dough. When it's evenly mixed, add the water gradually, mixing with your hands as you go, and kneading it into a dough. When you have a ball, it's ready to press into your large flan tin. Press it on the bottom and up the sides to make a shell. Don't make it too thick—if you have too much, reserve it and eat it as it is or make it into biscuits and dehydrate it. Store the crust in the fridge until you're ready to fill it. To make the filling, remove the flesh from the avocados and put it straight in the blender. Add in all the remaining ingredients and blend for a minute until you have a thick cream. Spoon it into the crust, and put it back in the fridge for a couple of hours to set.

Superbliss Tart

Serves ten
1 hour, 2 hours setting
Blender

One day I went swimming in the sea and thought I was going to die because I went too far out and couldn't get back. I loved it. I came home and made up this.

1 ¾ cups (175 g) almonds
1 ¾ cups (175 g) lucuma powder
4 Tbsp agave nectar
1 Tbsp cinnamon
½ cup (125 ml) water

⅔ cup (75 g) cacao butter
¾ cup (100 g) cacao nibs
3 (750 g) avocados
1 ¼ cups (125 g) mesquite powder
1 Tbsp (10 g) he shou wu
4 Tbsp agave nectar
1 cup (250 ml) water

To make the crust, grind up the almonds in a high-power blender. Transfer them to a mixing bowl, and add in the lucuma, stirring them together. Pour in the agave nectar and water, and mix by hand, kneading the dough into a ball. When it's firm, press into a large flan tin, and store in the fridge while you make the filling. Melt the cacao butter first. Grind the nibs in a high-power blender or coffee grinder. Slice open the avocados and spoon the flesh straight into your blender. Add in the nibs, mesquite, suma, agave nectar, melted butter and water—everything, in fact. Blend for a few minutes until you have a light brown cream with no bits of nib left. Spoon into the crust and leave in the fridge to set for two hours.

Jesus Loves You To Gojiness Tart

Serves ten
1 hour presoaking, 2 hours setting
Blender

> Jesus died for our sins, and this tart will do the same for you. Eat it and be redeemed.

Crust
1 ¼ cups (125 g) gojis
1 ¼ cups (125 g) oats
1 ¼ cups (125 g) lucuma powder
½ cup (125 ml) water

2 cups (200 g) gojis, soaked 1 hour
¾ cup (100 g) cacao butter
3 (750 g) avocados
1 cup (100 g) mesquite powder
2 lemons, juiced
3 Tbsp agave nectar
1 cup (250 ml) water

Make sure you've presoaked your gojis for the filling. To make the crust, grind up the unsoaked gojis into a flour in a grinder or high-power blender. Transfer them to a mixing bowl and then grind up the oats. Put the oats in the bowl with the gojis and lucuma and mix the flours together with your hands. Add the water gradually, kneading the dough into a ball as you do. When you have one single mass, press it into your flan tin, lining the sides and the base about ½ cm (¼") thick. If you have any left over you can make little cookies with it and dehydrate it.

To make the filling, melt the cacao butter first. Scoop the flesh out of the avocados and put it in the blender. Add in the mesquite, lemon juice, agave nectar, and gojis and blend to a cream. Keep blending and add the cacao butter gradually. Once you have a huge blob of orange smoothness, spoon it out into your flan tin. Pop in the fridge to set for a couple of hours. Will keep stored in the fridge for up to two weeks.

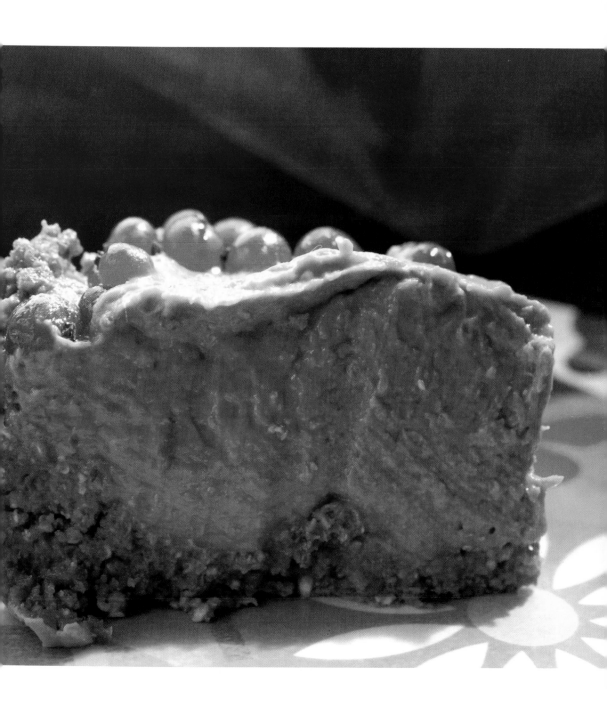

Rosemary's Rose Cheezecake

Serves eight
Needs three days at least to soak the Irish moss, then it will take you about 20 minutes to make the cake and another 2–3 hours to set it.
You also need a high-power blender

In honor of my dear friend Rosemary, who always inspires me to create something new and exciting in the kitchen when she comes over. This Irish moss-based dessert is so gorgeously light, you may need to weight your pockets down with stones after you've eaten it, to prevent you from floating up to the heavens.

Base
1 cup (100 g) buckwheaties
1 cup (90 g) almonds
2 Tbsp raw honey
½ cup (60 g) coconut oil

Topping
1 oz (30 g) Irish moss
2 cups (500 ml) water
1 cup (125 g) cashews
   presoaked 4–8 hours)
10 drops rose essential oil
2 tsp vanilla powder or
   1 vanilla pod
1 cup (125 g) coconut oil
½ cup (50 g) lucuma powder
4–8 Tbsp agave nectar
2 tsp ashwagandha powder
1 tsp Etherium Gold
Gojis to decorate

To make the base, grind the buckwheaties and almonds to a flour. Melt the coconut oil if necessary, and stir it into the flour with the honey. Press it into the base of a silicon mold (or cake tin lined with greaseproof paper or aluminum foil). Pop it in the fridge to set while you make the topping.

Prepare your Irish moss according to the given instructions. This is the method we have found works with the red moss that we have in Europe. If you are using the white kind, it may behave differently, so please check the manufacturer's instructions carefully to ensure the best results. If you get it wrong, your cake could turn out too runny or too firm. Take your moss and rinse it well. Then find an airtight container to house it in (we use our empty 1 kg coconut butter tubs), and put the moss and 1 cup (250 ml) pure water in the tub. Put the lid on and leave it in the fridge. We find our moss likes a minimum of three days soaking, and up to five days.

When you're ready to use it, throw away the soak water, and make sure NOT to rinse the moss again. Blend it up with 1 cup (250 ml) of the water. Blend it for a good few minutes until the moss is broken down as much as possible, and the mixture starts to go light and fluffy.

Add all the other ingredients into the blender: the cashews, rose, vanilla, coconut oil, lucuma, agave, ashwagandha and Etherium Gold. Blend for a good couple of minutes. I don't have much of a sweet tooth, so 4 Tbsp agave tastes perfect to me, but if you do love the sugary sweet stuff, you may want to up the agave to as much as eight tablespoons. Add the second cup of water (250 ml), and blend again until it's light and fluffy.

Pour it out over the buckwheat base and leave to set in the fridge for at least two hours. When it's set, it should be light and moussey, but firm enough to slice. Decorate with handfuls of goji berries, or fresh berries such as strawberries if they are in season. Will keep for up to a week in the fridge, if you can stop it floating off up to heaven.

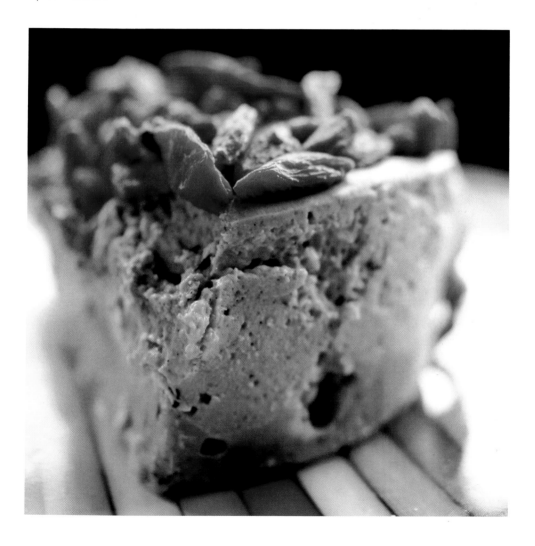

Matrix Tart

Serves 12
1 hour, 3 hours setting
Blender

OK, so this is like a deviant mince-meat tart. And when Zachary was only three years old he got *The Matrix* and mincemeat confused, as you do when you're three. But it actually fits because the apples and berries do make a kind of criss-cross matrix pattern. So see? Sometimes things that seem really silly at the time end up making perfect sense. Or sometimes the things that you thought made sense are actually nonsense.

Crust
1 ¼ cups (125 g) goji berries
½ cup (60 g) cacao powder
1 ¼ cups (125 g) almonds
½ cup (60 g) lucuma powder
½ cup (125 ml) water

1 lb (500 g) apples
2 ½ cups (250 g) goji berries
½ cup (50 g) dried cranberries
½ cup (50 g) dried barberries *
½ cup (50 g) dried mulberries
1 cup (100 g) pine nuts
2 (500 g) avocados
2 Tbsp flax oil
1 lemon, juiced
1 Tbsp honey
1 Tbsp cinnamon
1 Tbsp psyllium

To make the crust, grind the gojis into flour in a high-power blender or grinder. Transfer them to a mixing bowl, and add in the cacao powder, almonds, and lucuma. Roll up your sleeves, and mix it up with your hands. Add in the water a little at a time, kneading as you go, so you end up with a firm ball of dough. Press it into your flan tin, lining the sides and the bottom with a layer about ½ cm (¼") thick. Any leftovers you can eat!

To make the filling, grate the apples and put them in a large mixing bowl with the gojis, cranberries, barberries, mulberries, and pine nuts. If you can't get hold of one or more of these berries, you can always substitute raisins or chopped dried apricots or dates. Put everything else in a blender: the avocado flesh, lemon juice, flax oil, honey, and cinnamon. Blend to a thick cream, then add in the psyllium and give it another quick blitz. Spoon your avocado mix into your apple mix and stir it all together, making sure all your apple is coated in avocado. Spoon it into your flan tin and press it down. Pop in the fridge for a couple of hours to firm up. Serve with cream—Maca'd Up, Super Hemp Cream Me, or Angels are Delighted, whatever you like as long as it doesn't have cows in.

* Available at rawliving.eu

Cacao Crunch Cake

Serves 12
1 hour, 3 hours setting
Blender

So here's the true story of this cake. When I was 20, I had a bad trip on Brighton Beach and when I was coming down the next day I ate a whole cake I had made, a vegan fridge cake with carob and broken biscuit crumbs and lots of sweetness. It tasted wonderful while I was eating it, but then I felt really sick, so I had some chips cos I needed something savory, and then I felt even more sick and fat and not very happy. But the taste of that fridge cake haunted me, and when we moved to Brighton in 2005 I kept remembering it. I tried to recreate it, and this is the end result. A lot of people have said to me it's the best cake they've ever eaten. But if I hadn't had that bad trip, I'd never have come up with it 15 years later. Funny how things work, isn't it?

1 ¾ cups (220 g) coconut oil
2 cups (250 g) cacao nibs
2 cups (200 g) lucuma powder
1 cup (100 g) mesquite powder
1 Tbsp purple corn extract
2 ½ cups (250 g) Raw Living Hi-trail*

Icing
1 cup (125 g) cacao butter
1 cup (125 g) shelled hemp seeds
½ cup (60 g) mesquite powder
½ cup (125 ml) water
1 tsp purple corn extract

Melt the coconut oil to start. Grind up the nibs in a high-power blender or grinder. In a large mixing bowl, stir together the nibs, lucuma, mesquite and purple corn extract. Once it's evenly mixed, add in your Hi-trail. Then pour in your melted butter and mix it in to a sloppy goo. Pour it into a cake tin and leave to set in the fridge.

To make the icing, begin by melting the cacao butter. Once it's liquid, put it in the blender with the remaining ingredients. Blend to a cream, making sure the hemp seeds are fully blended in and the cream is not bitty. At this stage it will be quite runny. Spread on top of your cake, and it will set in 2–3 hours. When ready it should be firm, though still soft.

*Available at rawliving.eu or find equivalent. Hi-Trail is a trail mix made of sprouted and dried seeds, vine fruit, goji berries and 30% cacao nibs.

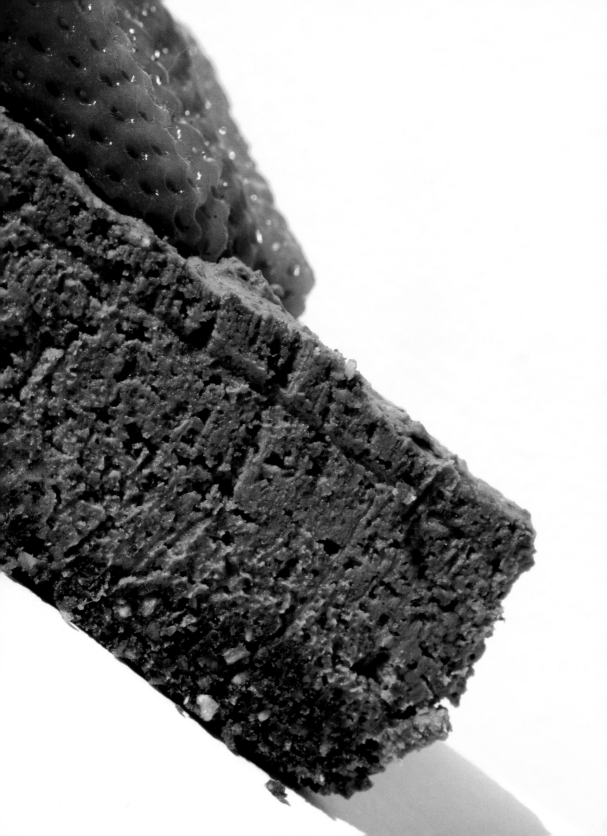

Blissberry Tart

Serves 12
1 hour, 3 hours setting
Blender

Berries and chocolate are a supersexy combination. Cherries are brilliant, if you can be bothered to sit and stone them. Blueberries are heavenly, if you can afford them. Or mix 'em up—strawberries and raspberries together are beautiful.

Crust
1 ¼ cups (125 g) oats
1 ¼ cups (125 g) almonds
½ cup (60 g) lucuma powder
½ cup (60 g) cacao powder
½ cup (125 ml) water

¾ cup (100 g) cacao butter
2 cups (250 g) cacao nibs
4 cups (500 g) strawberries,
   blueberries, cherries or
   raspberries
1 (250 g) avocado
1 cup (100 g) mesquite powder
½ cup (75 g) xylitol
1 Tbsp purple corn extract

To make the crust, grind the oats to flour in a grinder or high-power blender. Transfer them to a mixing bowl and grind up the almonds. Put the almonds in the bowl with the oats and add in the lucuma and cacao powder. Give it all a good mix together with your clean hands. Add the water little by little, mixing with your hands and pressing the dough together to make a ball. Press into your flan tin, lining the sides and bottom with a layer about ½ cm (¼ ") thick. Any leftovers, roll into balls and eat. Put the case in the fridge while you make the filling.

Melt the cacao butter first. Grind up the cacao nibs in a grinder or high-power blender. Remove any extraneous stems etc. from the berries, and put them in the blender. Scoop the flesh out of the avocado and put that in too. Put the nibs and butter in, along with the mesquite, xylitol and purple corn extract, and give it all a good blend for a couple of minutes until you have a thick cream. Spoon it into your pastry case, and leave it in the fridge to set for a couple of hours more. Will keep in the fridge for up to one week.

Cosmic Cacao Cake

Serves 10
1 hour, 3 hours setting
Blender

> This was our most popular cake in the Raw Magic shop. You can vary it with any nut or seed to replace the sesame. If you can't be bothered to make it yourself, we also sell this one online in lots of different incarnations.

2 cups (250 g) sesame seeds
2 cups (250 g) cacao nibs
2 cups (200 g) lucuma powder
⅔ cup (90 g) xylitol or coconut sugar
1 cup (250 ml) water

Icing
2 (500 g) avocados
¼ cup (30 g) cacao powder
2 Tbsp agave nectar
1 Tbsp mucuna
2 Tbsp bee pollen
2 Tbsp shelled hemp seeds

Grind the sesame seeds up in a high-power blender or grinder. Transfer them to a large mixing bowl. Grind the nibs up in the same way, and put them in the bowl too. Add the lucuma and xylitol in and give it all a good stir so it's evenly mixed. Pour in the water and stir it in so you have a thick cookie mixture. Spoon it into a cake tin and pop in the fridge to set for three hours.

Once it's ready, you can make your icing. Peel the avocados, spoon out the flesh and put them in the blender. Add the cacao powder, agave nectar and suma and blend it all together to a cream. Spoon over the top and sides of the cake, so it covers the whole cake evenly. Decorate the top with the bee pollen and hemp seeds.

Hi-Cake

Makes 8 large slices
30 mins, 3 hours setting time
Blender

We started selling the Hi-bar in April 2005, the first raw chocolate bar to be sold in the UK, and possibly the world. For some reason, we found it really hard to find good bar molds, so for about six months we just had one single mold that the oompa loompas would press the chocolate into and turn out. We've got it framed on the wall of our kitchen now. This is the Hi-bar in a cake, made with cacao nibs and Brazil nuts.

Cake
2 cups (250 g) cacao nibs
2 cups (250 g) Brazil nuts
2 ½ cups (250 g) lucuma powder
6 Tbsp agave nectar
⅔ cup (150 ml) water

Icing
2 (500 g) avocados
⅓ cup (30 g) cacao powder
2 Tbsp agave nectar
¼ cup (60 ml) water

Decoration
2 Tbsp goji berries
2 Tbsp dried cranberries

Grind up the nibs and nuts separately in a high-power blender or coffee grinder. Transfer to a mixing bowl with the lucuma and agave nectar. With your hands, mix the all the ingredients so you have an even powder. Add the water gradually, kneading the mixture into a ball with your hands. It should end up as a fairly thick dough-like consistency. Press into a springform cake tin or silicon mold and leave in the fridge to set for a few hours.

To make the icing, put the avocado flesh in the blender along with the cacao powder, agave nectar and water. If you haven't got cacao powder, you can substitute carob or mesquite. Blend until you have a thick cream. Once your cake is set, you can remove it from the cake tin, and spoon the icing evenly over the top and the sides. Decorate with dried goji berries and cranberries sprinkled over the top. Uneaten cake can be stored in an airtight container in the fridge for up to two weeks (but only if no one knows it's there).

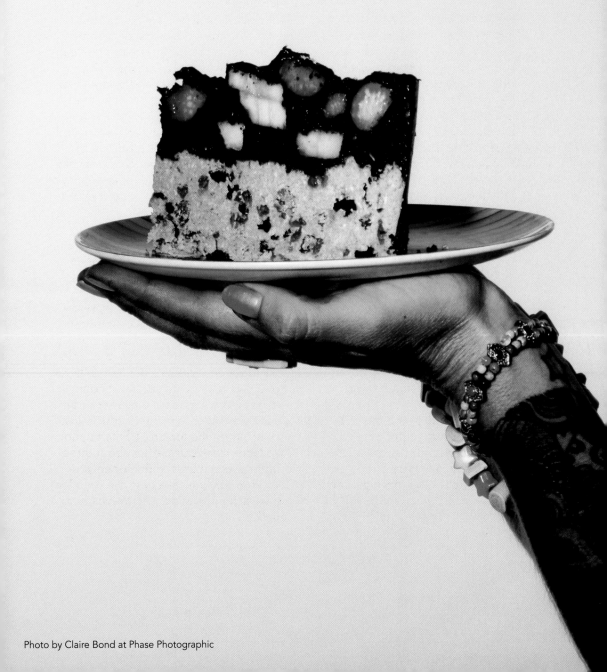

Photo by Claire Bond at Phase Photographic

King Zachary's Cake

Serves 12
1 hour, 3 hours setting
Blender

What else would a little boy want for his cake on his fourth birthday but one made with berries and honey? And where else would he want to go but Legoland, and what else would he dress up as but a King? Truly, my children lead a dream life. Cake and Lego—I know how to treat them like the Kings that they are.

1 ¾ cups (200 g) cacao butter
2 cups (200 g) buckwheaties (p. 80)
1 cup (100 g) lucuma powder
½ cup (50 g) gojis
½ cup (50 g) dried mulberries
½ cup (50 g) dried barberries*
½ cup (50 g) dried cranberries
   (apple juice sweetened)
½ cup (100 g) honey
1 cup (250 ml) water

Icing
2 cups (250 g) strawberries
1 banana
1 ¾ cup (200 g) coconut oil
⅓ cup (50 g) xylitol or
   coconut palm sugar
4 Tbsp agave nectar
1 ¾ cup (175 g) cacao powder

Melt the cacao butter first. Grind the buckwheaties into flour in a grinder or high-power blender. In a mixing bowl, stir together the buckwheat flour and lucuma. Then add in the gojis, mulberries, barberries and cranberries. If you can't get hold of one or more of these berries, you can substitute with extra gojis or raisins. Stir them in, then pour in your honey and water, and blend to a runny dough using your hands or a spoon. Pop the dough into a springform cake tin and transfer to the fridge to start setting.

Start making the icing by melting the coconut oil. Prepare the strawberries and banana by chopping them into large bite-sized chunks. In a mixing bowl, pop in the cacao powder, xylitol, and agave nectar, and give it a good mix. Stir in the oil, and when you've got a runny chocolate cream, stir in the bananas and strawberries. Pour this mix over the top of your cake, so it forms a thick top layer about a quarter of the size of the cake mixture—it should just sit nicely on the top and fill the tin, not spill down the sides. After about three hours, when it's set, spring open your tin and slide the cake out. Will keep for a week if the kids don't know where to find it.

*Available at rawliving.eu

Cake Mates

Serves 16
1 hour, 3 hours setting
Blender

A cake mate is like a soul mate but better, someone with whom you can have your cake and eat it, someone who you worship and who worships you back. If you're not up for what is, quite honestly, a pretty tripped-out cake, you can make it without all the extra added superfoods.

Base
1 ¾ cup (200 g) coconut oil
1 cup (100 g) buckwheaties (p. 78)
1 cup (100 g) maca
1 cup (100 g) lucuma powder
1 Tbsp suma
1 tsp Etherium Gold
⅓ cup (50 g) xylitol

Chocolate layer
2 cups (240 g) cacao butter
1 ½ cups (150 g) cacao powder
2 cups (200 g) mesquite powder
2 Tbsp Crystal Manna or
    E3 AFA flakes
1 tsp Etherium Black

Topping
3 (750 g) avocados
¾ cup (100 g) shelled hemp seeds
½ cup agave nectar
1 Tbsp purple corn extract
1 tsp Etherium Pink

Decoration
2 Tbsp goji berries
2 Tbsp bee pollen
2 Tbsp shelled hemp seeds

To make the base, first melt the coconut oil. Grind the buckwheaties into flour in your blender or grinder, and then transfer them to a mixing bowl. Add the maca, lucuma, suma, gold and xylitol and mix the powders together with your hands. Once they're well mixed, pour in the coconut oil, and stir it up with a spoon. Transfer immediately to a large flan dish, and press down flat with a spoon. Pop in the fridge to help it set.

Next make the chocolate. Melt the cacao butter to start. In a mixing bowl, put your cacao powder, mesquite, Crystal Manna and Etherium Black and stir them together with a spoon. Once the butter's melted, stir that in too. Remove the base from the fridge, and pour the chocolate layer on top. Put it back in the fridge. If you've got time, you may want to wait a couple of hours before making the next layer, to give the chocolate time to set.

To make the topping, remove the flesh from the avocados and transfer to the blender. Put in all the other ingredients and blend together to a thick purple cream. Remove the cake from the fridge, and spoon the avocado mixture over the top. Decorate with the gojis, hemp and pollen in concentric circles. Any leftovers will keep in the fridge for up to a week, but only if you put an invisible protection spell over it so no one can see it.

Candies and Spreads

Believe it or not, sometimes you want a sweet snack that isn't chocolate.

Sometimes chocolate just won't cut the custard, and that's where these little babies come in. We've got lots of candy, some trail mixes, and some creams for spreading on crackers, using as cake icings, pouring over fruit, or just over your best friend. In fact, pour them over anybody you take a fancy to, and if they're not your best friend already, then they soon will be.

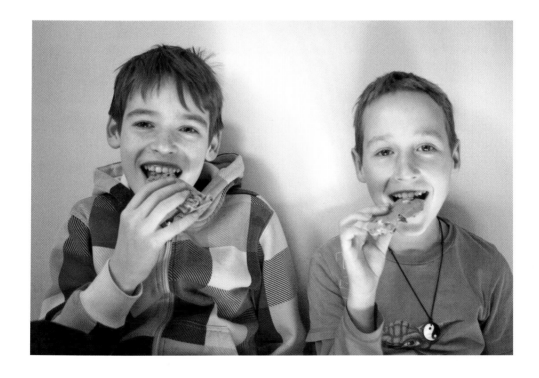

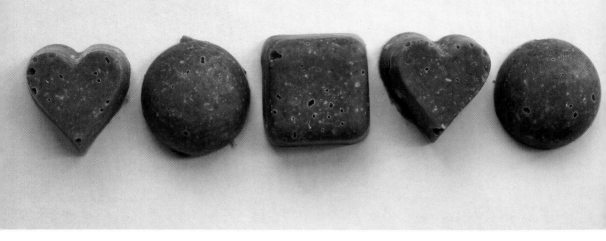

Fudging Awesome

Makes 16 pieces
10 mins, 2–3 hours setting
Blender

Everyone loves gojis, and everyone loves goji fudge. And be warned, everyone eats too much of this when they first try it.

1 ¼ cups (150 g) coconut oil
1 cup (100 g) gojis
3 Tbsp agave nectar
¾ cup (75 g) mesquite powder
¾ cup (75 g) lucuma powder

Melt the coconut oil first. Pour it in a high-power blender with the gojis and agave nectar. Blend for a few minutes. They won't form a cream, but the gojis will break down into a mass. It's tricky to get it right—if you blend too long, the oil in the gojis will start to separate, if you don't blend long enough your end result will not be smooth. Add the mesquite and lucuma and blend again; this time it should make a cream. Pour into a small tray and leave it to set in the fridge for 2–3 hours. Once it's hard, cut into 16 pieces.

Crystal Omega Fudge

Makes 30 pieces
10 mins, 2 hours setting
Blender

> You can also try this with pumpkin butter, or in fact any nut butter that tickles your taste buds.

1 ¼ cups (150 g) coconut oil
1 cup (150 g) hemp butter
1 cup (100 g) mesquite powder
1 cup (100 g) maca
3 Tbsp agave nectar
2 Tbsp Crystal Manna
   or E3 AFA flakes

Melt the coconut oil first. In a blender, blend the melted coconut with the hemp butter to a liquid. Then add the mesquite, maca and agave nectar and blend again. Stir in the Crystal Manna and pour into a large tray. Set in the fridge for 2–3 hours. Turn out and cut into cubes, five across by six down.

Golden Goji Love

Makes 25 squares
10 mins, 2 hours setting
Blender

> We use the heart-shaped silicon molds for these, they are a pretty essential piece of kit when it comes to making candies and chocolates. I use my oven for storing my silicon molds and I must have around 20 different kinds: hearts, shells, arrows, the alphabet, space invaders, gingerbread men, miniature cupcakes...there are an infinite number available in the shops and they make sweet-making so much more fun, especially when you're making them as presents.

1 ¼ cups (150 g) cacao butter
1 cup (100 g) goji berries
3 Tbsp agave nectar
1 cup (100 g) lucuma powder
1 tsp Etherium Gold

Start by melting the cacao butter. Put the goji berries in a high-power blender or grinder, and grind to a powder. It doesn't have to be too fine, just as long as there are no whole berries left. Add the agave nectar and melted butter in and blend again to a liquid. Then add the lucuma and Gold in and briefly blend one more time. Do not over-blend or the oil from the gojis will start to separate. Pour into molds and leave for at least two hours to set. When they're ready, pop them out, and remember, these are for SHARING.

It's the Buzzness

Makes 25 pieces
10 mins, 3 hours setting
No equipment needed

> Everyone loves this candy; it's a perfect pick-me-up. Bee pollen and purple corn extract are a winning team, purple keeps you focused while the pollen keeps you moving.

1 ¼ cups (150 g) coconut oil
1 ½ cups (150 g) bee pollen
1 ½ cups (150 g) lucuma powder
½ tsp crystal salt
1 tsp purple corn extract

Melt the oil first. Once it's liquid, stir all the ingredients together in a bowl, and pour into a tray to set. Leave in the fridge for three hours, by which time it should be hard. Turn out and cut into cubes, five up by five down.

Macaculous Fudge

Makes 25 pieces
10 mins, 3 hours setting
Blender

> Cacao butter and lucuma is such a great combination in sweets—try our Raw Living Truth bar if you need convincing. This is packed with maca for extra energy.

¾ cup (100 g) cacao butter
1 cup (125 g) shelled hemp seeds
1 cup (100 g) maca
½ cup (50 g) lucuma powder
3 Tbsp agave nectar
1 tsp Aulterra

Melt the butter. Mash the hemp seeds to a paste in a blender or food grinder. Add the melted butter and blend again so you have a runny cream. Add in the remaining ingredients and blend one more time. Press into a tray, and leave in the fridge for three hours to set; you should have a solid but soft candy. When it's ready, turn out and cut into pieces, five by five. Keeps for up to a week in the fridge.

Fudge Me

Makes 16 pieces
15 mins, 2 hours setting
Blender

> We used to sell a lot of this in the Raw Magic shop. It's very filling, grounding and energizing without being overstimulating like chocolate can sometimes be.

1 ¾ cups (220 g) shelled hemp seeds
½ cup (50 g) mesquite powder
2 Tbsp agave nectar
1 tsp suma

Grind up the hemp seeds in a high-power blender or grinder. If you're using a high-power blender, add in the mesquite and agave nectar, otherwise transfer to a food processor and blend again. When you have a sticky mass, scrape it out with a spoon and press into a small tray. Leave it in the fridge to set for two hours. When it's ready, cut into cubes, four up by four down. Keeps for up to a week in the fridge.

Caramaca

Makes 16 pieces
10 mins, 3 hours setting
No equipment needed

> This was one of the first sweets we sold, originally known as Maca Bar. It's super-strengthening, and very more-ish, but unfortunately it doesn't keep well so we had to stop making it. Maca tastes a bit like sick when it goes rancid, which isn't what you want from a sweet treat really, is it? Be warned, most things made with maca are best eaten within 24 hours. Only if your recipe contains no water, only a little maca, lots of fat, and it doesn't leave the fridge, will you get away with it.

1 cup (100 g) maca
1 cup (100 g) mesquite powder
1 ¼ cup (150 g) coconut oil
1 Tbsp vanilla powder or
    1 Tbsp pure vanilla concentrate

Melt the coconut oil first. When it's liquid, transfer to a mixing bowl, and stir in the mesquite, maca and vanilla. Pour into a small tray, and leave in the fridge to set for 2–3 hours. When it's ready, turn out and cut into cubes, four across by four down. Keeps in the fridge for up to one week.

Camu Believe It

Makes 25 pieces
10 mins, 3 hours setting
Blender

> This is a gorgeously gentle candy, for when you actually don't feel like being energized, tripped out or shaken up much at all. Better make a double batch if you want to eat any yourself—this one disappears faster than you can say, "I only made that yesterday."

¾ cup (100 g) cacao butter
¾ cup (100 g) coconut oil
¾ cup (100 g) shelled hemp seeds
3 Tbsp agave nectar
1 cup (100 g) mesquite powder
1 cup (100 g) lucuma
2 Tbsp camu camu
1 Tbsp purple corn extract

Melt both butters together. Mash the hemp seeds up in a blender or grinder. Then blend them up with the melted butters. Add the remaining ingredients to the blender and blend one more time. Pour into a medium-sized tray and leave in the fridge to set for three hours. When it's hard, turn out and cut into cubes, five across by five down.

All That Glitters Is Not Green

Makes 25 pieces
10 mins, 3 hours setting
No equipment needed

> OK, I admit it, it's hard to make spirulina taste nice. A few people like it, but most people find it pretty hard to stomach. I've done my best here to cram algae into a sweet bar that tastes so yummy you'll keep eating it. Actually, one of the best reviews I had of the first edition of this book was when someone said, "She even manages to make Spirulina taste good!"

1 ½ cups (150 g) cacao butter
¾ cup (75 g) spirulina
½ cup (50 g) mesquite powder
½ cup (50 g) lucuma powder
1 Tbsp agave nectar
1 Tbsp Crystal Manna or
    E3 AFA flakes

Melt the cacao butter first. Once it's liquid, transfer to a mixing bowl, and stir in all the other ingredients, leaving ½ tbsp Crystal Manna aside. Give it all a good stir and pour into a medium-sized tray. Sprinkle on the remaining Crystal Manna, pressing it gently into the candy. Leave in the fridge to set for three hours. When it's ready, turn out carefully, trying not to lose any of the Crystal Manna from the top. Cut into cubes, five by five.

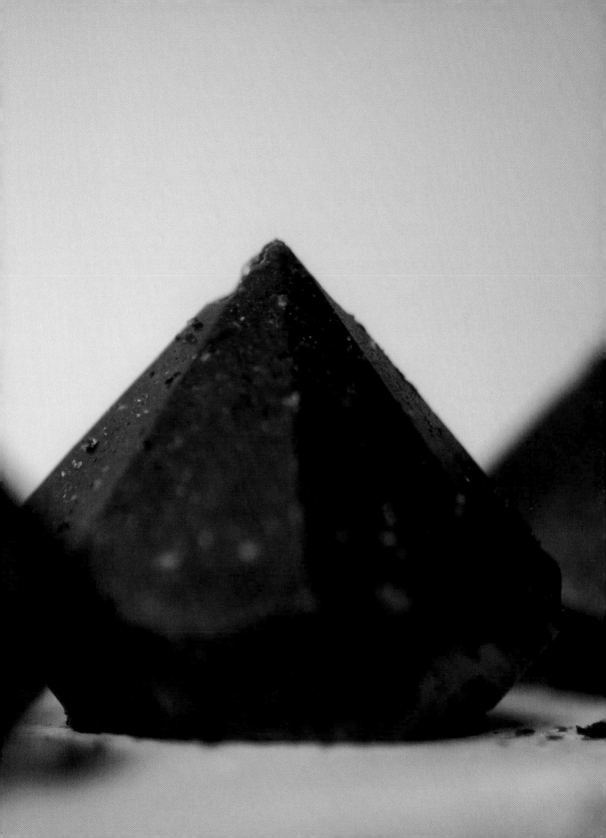

Mulberry Mud

Makes 20 pieces
15 mins, 3 hours setting
Blender

Mud, mud, glorious mud, there's nothing quite like it for cooling the blood. I can't actually say for sure that this candy will cool your blood, but it will do something to your body that could make you dance around the kitchen in a pleasant sort of muddy mulberry madness.

1 ¼ cups (150 g) cacao butter
2 cups (200 g) mulberries
1 cup (100 g) mesquite powder
1 tsp Etherium Red
1 Tbsp suma

Start off by melting the cacao butter. Blend the mulberries to a mash in the blender. Add the melted butter in and blend again to a liquid. Add the mesquite, Etherium Red, and suma in and blend one more time until you have a smooth cream. Pour into a medium-sized tray and leave to set in the fridge for three hours. When it's ready, turn it out and cut into cubes, five across by four down, 20 all together. Will keep stored in the fridge for a couple of weeks.

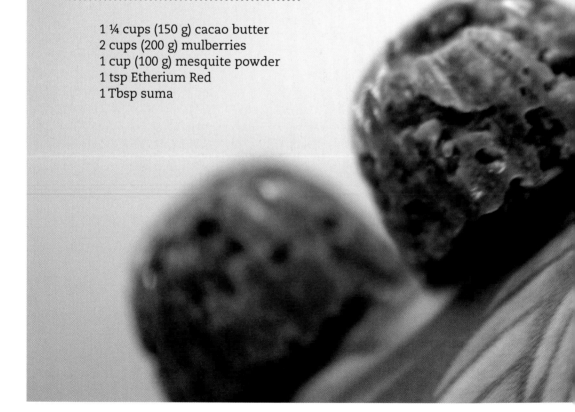

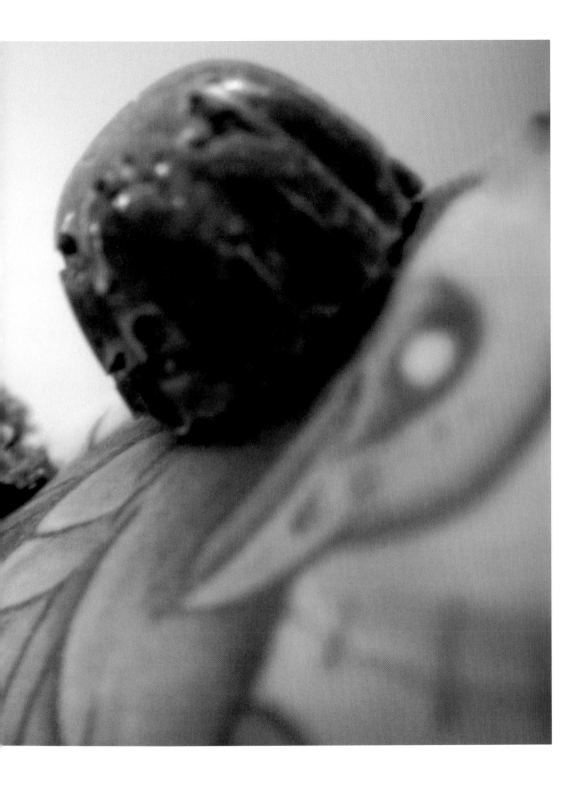

Super Hemp Cream Me

Serves eight
5 mins
Blender

This is gorgeous as a dip for fruit, perfect as an icing for cakes, or spread it on bread for a teatime snack.

2 cups (250 g) shelled hemp seeds
1 ¼ cups (125 g) lucuma powder
1 cup (90 g) xylitol
1 vanilla pod or
  1 Tbsp vanilla powder
1 cup (250 ml) water

Put all the ingredients in the blender together and blend for a couple of minutes until you have a thick cream. Keeps in the fridge for up to a week. It will thicken when stored, so you may want to add a little extra water.

Right Said Fred Spread

Serves six
5 mins
No equipment needed

Remember them? If this spread could sing it would go, "I'm too sexy, I'm too sexy for this recipe book." Deadly simple, deadly effective, deadly delicious, spread this on anything if you are ready to die and go to heaven.

3 Tbsp cacao powder
2 Tbsp almond butter
  (white if available)
2 Tbsp flax oil
2 Tbsp raw honey
1 tsp suma

Put everything in a large bowl and mix with a spoon. Store in the fridge, it will keep for a couple of weeks.

Maca'd Up

Serves four
5 mins
No equipment needed

> This is so beautifully quick and simple to make, goes lovely on bread (pages 186–188), and is a nice easy way to make sure you get your maca in you.

4 Tbsp maca powder
4 Tbsp raw tahini
4 Tbsp agave nectar
4 Tbsp hemp oil
1 cup (250 ml) pure water

Spoon it all into a bowl apart from the water. With a small spoon, give it a good stir. The maca is very absorbent and your mixture will go very dry and stiff (you can just eat it like this if you're feeling piggy! Or roll it into walnut-sized balls to make little sweeties). Add the water, a tablespoon at a time, until you reach the desired consistency, runny like tahini. The end result should be sweet, rich, creamy, and utterly irresistible.

Angels Are Delighted

Serves four
15 mins
Blender

> This cream will transport even the most depraved and sinful of you to heaven immediately.

1 avocado
¾ cup (100 g) shelled hemp seeds
2 Tbsp camu camu
¾ cup (75 g) xylitol or
    coconut palm sugar
1 cup (250 ml) water

Remove the flesh from the avocado and scoop it into the blender. Add in the hemp seeds, camu camu and xylitol and blend to a cream. With the blender running, add the water gradually. Store in the fridge, will keep for up to a week.

Love Butter

Makes one large tub
15 mins
Blender

> No ifs, no buts, just love.

2 cups (250 g) shelled hemp seeds
¾ cup (75 g) cacao powder
½ cup (50 g) maca powder
4 Tbsp raw honey
1 tsp white miso
2 Tbsp hemp oil
1 ½ cups (350 ml) water

Put everything in the blender apart from the water. Mash up the hemp seeds a bit then gradually add the water, keeping the blender running as you go. Give it a minute or two, then it's ready. Keeps in the fridge, although keep it away from things that go off easily—this butter is HOT.

Matchmake Me

Makes one jar
10 mins
Blender

> Cheeky and minty, as you stir this, visualize your perfect chocolate boyfriend or girlfriend and then when you meet them, you will know it was all down to eating this spread on bread (pages 186–188) at 2:30 every day for afternoon tea, and you can write and thank me, and send me pictures showing how beautiful you look together.

¾ cup (100 g) coconut oil
¾ cup (100 g) shelled hemp seeds
½ cup (50 g) xylitol or
    coconut sugar
5 drops peppermint oil
¼ cup (60 ml) water

Melt the coconut oil first. Mash the hemp seeds in the blender, then add the melted butter and blend again. Add in the xylitol and peppermint oil and keep the blender turning while you add the water gradually. Once it's done, you can eat it like this as a runny cream over fruit, or leave it in the fridge to harden into more of a spread.

Purple Love Cream

Makes four servings
5 mins
No equipment needed

> Have your way with this cream. Spread it on bread, use it as a fondant center in chocolate-making, dip strawberries in it, or cover someone you love in it and lick it off. Yum....

3 Tbsp agave nectar
¼ cup (50 g) raw tahini
2 tsp purple corn extract
2 tsp liquid maca extract
5 drops rose essential oil

Mix everything together in a bowl with a spoon to form a paste. Store in the fridge. Keeps well.

Barleypear

Serves four
5 mins, 12 hours drying
Blender, dehydrator

> This is a brilliant way to get the alkalizing greens into kids, or yourself; they make perfect snacks to put into packed lunches. You can also make the same recipe with spirulina and apple.

2 large (500 g) pears
1 Tbsp barleygrass powder

Remove the stems from the pears. Slice them into pieces to fit comfortably into your blender, removing cores and seeds. Put them in the blender with the barleygrass and whiz for a few minutes until there are no lumps of pear left. Spread over drying sheets and dry for 12 hours. When they're leathery and there are no moist bits left, remove them, and tear into strips. Store in an airtight container, they will keep for several weeks.

Space Dust

Serves four
5 mins
No equipment needed

> This makes a joyous sprinkle for cereal, yogurt, cake toppings, salad—anything that could do with a little extra joy, in short. It kind of tingles in your mouth and brightens up your life.

4 Tbsp bee pollen
4 Tbsp shelled hemp seeds
4 Tbsp cacao nibs
2 Tbsp raisins

Mix! You can even just eat it straight as it is, it's perfect for when you're on the go and don't have time to eat anything.

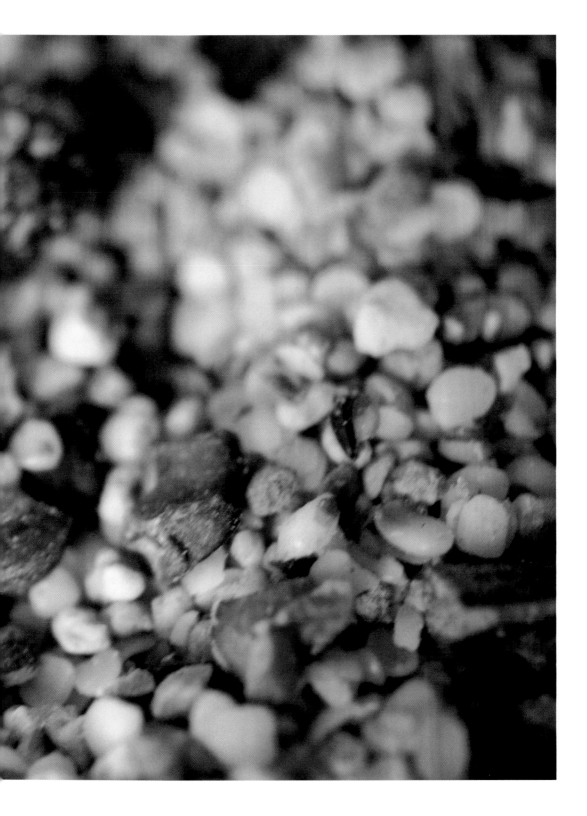

Super Super Trail

Serves four
5 mins
No equipment needed

> Another super easy, super energizing trail mix to add to anything and everything and spread a little super superness.

    ½ cup (50 g) goji berries
    ½ cup (25 g) coconut flakes
    ½ cup (50 g) cacao nibs
    ¼ cup (25 g) raisins
    ¼ cup (25 g) bee pollen

And…mix! And…eat!

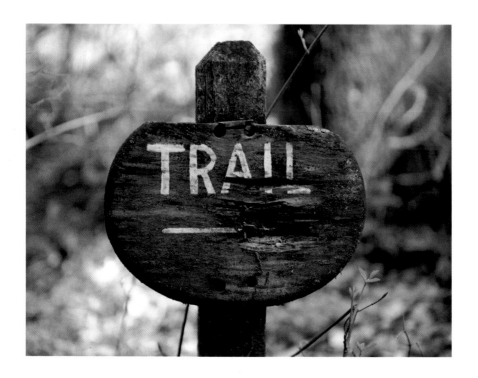

Chocolate

OK, well you know what?
I think this book is worth
the cover price for these
chocolate recipes alone.

We were fortunate to be among the first people in the UK to be introduced to the wonders of raw chocolate, and since then I have spent many hours in the kitchen experimenting with the alchemical wonders of cacao. It has become a staple part of our diet, and the many people who live and pass through our household eat it on a daily basis. How many mothers try and make sure their children eat their chocolate every day?! I always lace it with superfoods, so as well as the extraordinary nutritional content of the cacao, we are getting extras like algae, bee pollen, maca and goji berries. The Etheriums also work really well in chocolate. Where I have included Etheriums in the recipes, you can always omit them if you don't have access to them; it won't affect the taste. And you can also add them into any recipe if you feel drawn to do so. So here are a few of my favorite recipes, born out of testing over and over again what works (it's a hard job, eating chocolate every day!). And remember, chocolate-making is therapy, and above all, chocolate-making is fun. So use your imagination, be intuitive, and let yourself go wild in the kitchen creating your own alchemical cacao creations.

I generally put a pinch of Himalayan crystal salt in my chocolate recipes—it improves the flavor and aids mineral absorption. Just an eighth of a teaspoon is enough in a batch of chocolate. I haven't mentioned it in the recipes, but if you have some on hand it's a good idea to include it. For a tray to pour it into, I use silicon molds, as I mentioned in the candies section. One last tip: if you're using a blender, when you've scraped the chocolate out of the blender jug, pour in a cup of pure freshly boiled water, and give it another blend. This will help clean the jug, but better than that, the resulting liquid is the most gorgeous creamy hot chocolate drink you have ever tasted.

Wherever possible, I would measure the ingredients out for chocolate-making using scales—it's much more accurate, and whereas for most raw cuisine 10 g here or there doesn't generally make much difference, chocolate-making is a bit more of a science, and it's best to be as spot-on as you can be. In all my other recipes, I generally work with measuring cups, but with chocolate I am more inclined to use scales.

Most chocolates will keep in the fridge for up to eight weeks unless otherwise stated in the recipe, but it is highly unlikely you will ever have to worry about that.

Instructions for melting coconut oil and cacao butter are on page 78. If you're in a warm climate, you won't need to melt the coconut oil as it will already be liquid at room temperature.

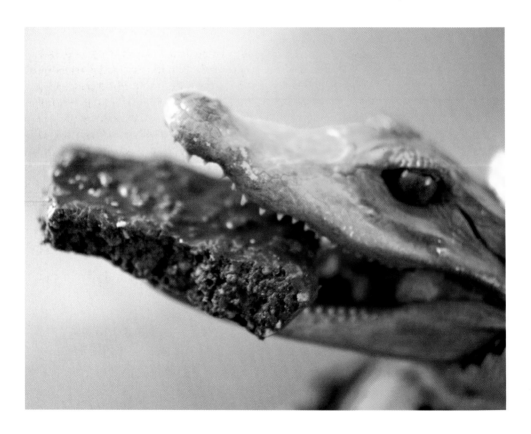

Oh My Goji

Serves 16
10 mins
Blender

> I was trying to make a spread with gojis and coconut oil, but it wasn't working. So I added some chocolate powder, came up with this, and took it over to a friend's house. That's one of the things about raw chocolate making—it's very, very hard to get it wrong, because even if it doesn't go to plan, it always ends up tasting the best ever.

1 ¼ cups (150 g) coconut oil
1 cup (100 g) goji berries
3 Tbsp agave nectar
1 ½ cups (150 g) cacao powder
½ cup (50 g) mesquite powder

Melt the coconut oil first, and once it's ready, put all the ingredients in the blender together and blend until there are no chips of goji left, and you have a thick cream. Pour into a small tray about 25 cm square, and leave in the fridge for three hours to set. Once it is ready, cut into 16 pieces.

Star Bar

Makes 36 pieces
15 mins, 3 hours setting
Blender

> Be the star that you really are! This one's such a winner, I wanted to make it into a bar, but the pollen doesn't keep well once it's ground up.

1 ½ cups (200 g) coconut oil
1 ½ cups (150 g) cacao powder
1 ½ cups (150 g) gojis
1 ½ cups (150 g) bee pollen
3 Tbsp agave nectar
2 tsp purple corn extract

Melt the oil first. Grind the cacao in a high-power blender or food grinder, and remove. Put the goji berries and pollen in the blender or grinder, and grind them up. Then add everything to the blender—melted butter, ground nibs, gojis and pollen, agave nectar, and purple corn extract. Blend again, until you have a thick gloop. Pour into a large tray, and leave in the fridge to set for three hours. When it's hard, cut into pieces, six across by six down. Will keep for up to five days in the fridge.

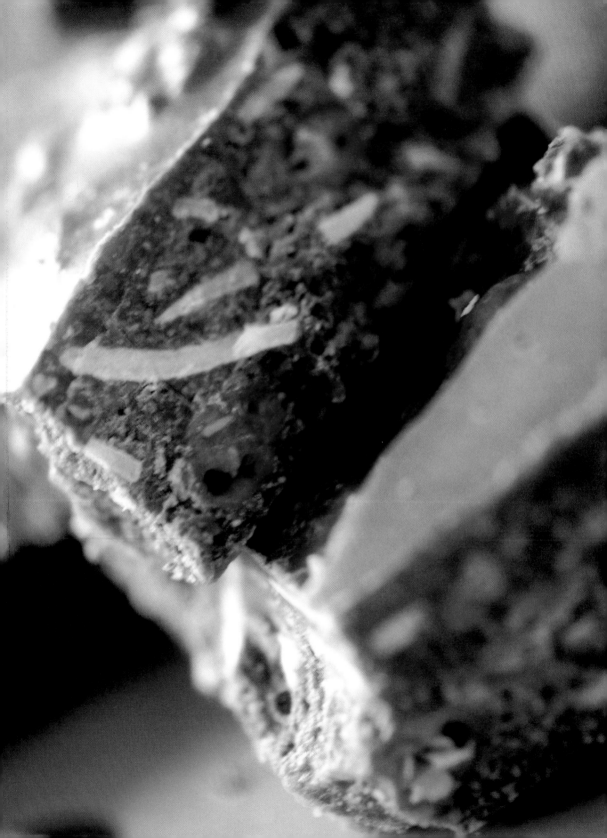

Goco Choco

Makes 36 pieces
15 mins, 3 hours setting
Blender

Grinding up gojis into your chocolate mixtures makes amazing results. Gojis have a naturally healthy low-glycemic sweetness which means you don't have to add so many powders and syrups to your chocolate mix. Coconut chips in chocolate are really beautiful; when you slice through the slab they make divine patterns.

1 ¾ cups (220 g) coconut oil
1 ½ cups (200 g) cacao nibs
1 ½ cups (150 g) goji berries
1 ½ cups (150 g) mesquite powder
3 Tbsp agave nectar
1 cup (50 g) coconut flakes
1 tsp Etherium Red

Melt the butter first. Grind up the nibs with ½ cup (50 g) gojis in a high-power blender or grinder. When fully ground, add in the butter and agave nectar and blend again for a minute. Once it's amalgamated, add the mesquite and Etherium Red and blend one more time. Stir in the remaining 1 cup (100 g) gojis and the coconut flakes by hand. I usually do this in the blender jug, but you can transfer to a bowl if you find it easier. Spoon into a tray and leave to set in the fridge for three hours. Once it's set, turn out and cut into pieces, six across by six down. Will keep in the fridge for up to eight weeks.

Siriusly Black

Makes 36 pieces
10 mins, 3 hours setting
Blender

Etherium Black and spirulina is a very grounding combination to keep you focused. I often use xylitol in my raw chocolate recipes. It is made from fermented birch bark and is a natural sugar substitute. It is very sweet, so you only need about half the amount you would use of the powders like mesquite or lucuma. It is good to add when you need some extra sweetness but don't want to add any more bulk to the recipe.

1 ¾ cups (220 g) coconut oil
2 cups (250 g) cacao nibs
1 cup (100 g) mesquite powder
½ cup (50 g) xylitol
1 tsp Etherium Black
½ cup (50 g) Spirulina

Melt the butter to start. Grind the nibs in a high-power blender*. Add the melted butter to the blender and blend again for a minute. Add in the remaining ingredients and blend one more time. Pour into a tray to set and leave in the fridge for three hours. Once it's set, pop out of the tray and cut into pieces, six down by six across.

*You can use a coffee grinder to grind the nibs, but will have to transfer to a blender for the remaining steps.

Pollen Put the Kettle On

Makes 36 pieces
10 mins, 3 hours setting
No equipment needed

Mmm, mulberries. Everyone who comes across them loves these sweet little Iranian berries. Sometimes they are quite crunchy, a bit like sugar puffs, but we like them best when they are moist and chewy and taste like honey. The softness of the mulberries contrasts beautifully with the crunchiness of the pollen. When we had the Raw Magic shop, we used to make dozens of different chocolate combinations and this was one of the most popular.

1 cup (110 g) coconut oil
1 cup (110 g) cacao butter
1 ½ cups (150 g) cacao powder
1 cup (100 g) lucuma powder
1 cup (100 g) mesquite powder
1 cup (100 g) mulberries
1 cup (100 g) bee pollen

Melt the coconut oil and cacao butter together. Cacao butter takes slightly longer to melt so put that in first. In a separate bowl, put your cacao powder, lucuma and mesquite, and stir together. Pour in the melted butters and stir again. Finally, add the mulberries and pollen and give them a good mix in. Pour the mixture into a large tray, and leave in the fridge to set for three hours. Once it's set, turn out and cut into cubes, six across by six down.

Maca Swirl

Makes 42 pieces
10 mins
No equipment needed

This is perhaps the most beautiful-looking recipe in the section. The marble effect is easy to do and so professional-looking. If you're a spirulina lover, you can make a green swirl by replacing the maca with spirulina.

1 ¼ cups (150 g) coconut oil
1 cup (100 g) cacao butter
1 ½ cups (150 g) cacao powder
1 cup (100 g) mesquite powder
1 cup (100 g) maca
½ cup (50 g) xylitol

For the swirl
¾ cup (100 g) coconut oil
¾ cup (80 g) lucuma powder
¾ cup (80 g) maca

Melt the coconut oil and cacao butter together. Cacao butter takes a little longer to melt, so put that in first. In a separate bowl, measure out the cacao powder, mesquite, maca and xylitol. Give them a good mix together, then pour in the butters and mix completely. In your heating bowl, heat the coconut oil for the swirl while you're mixing the chocolate. Then blend the oil, lucuma and maca in a bowl by hand. Pour half your chocolate into a large tray. Then pour some maca butter on top and swirl it around a bit, so it's creating patterns in the chocolate. Pour some more chocolate on top, then some more maca and keep going until you've used all the chocolate, but you need to keep half the maca for the top. With the rest of the maca butter, swirl it over the top of the chocolate, creating artistic patterns. You can drag it with a knife to create lines like a fancy cake. Leave to set in the fridge for three hours. When it's set, cut into pieces, seven across by six down. You will have gorgeous marble patterns running through the slab.

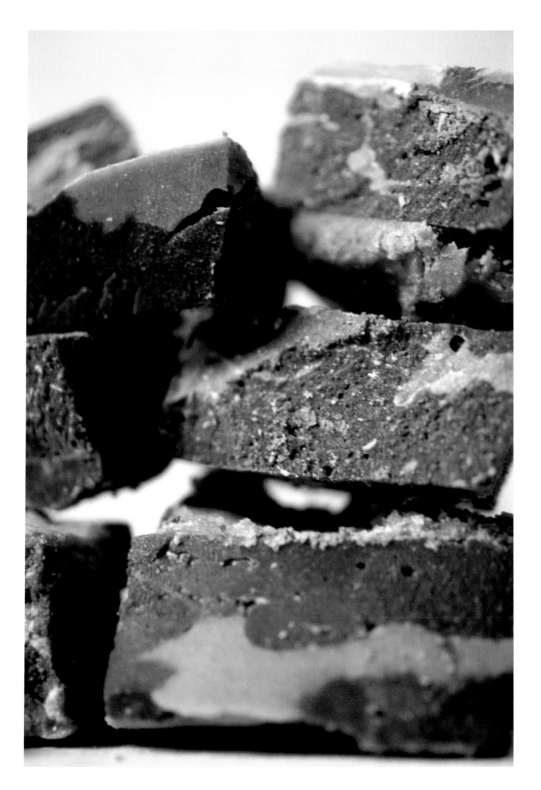

Suma Luvin

Makes 30 pieces
10 mins, 3 hours setting
No equipment needed

> Suma can make you feel like you're floating on a fluffy cloud, and when you mix it with Etherium Pink then it becomes a pink fluffy cloud and you feel in love with yourself, your life, your world, the earth, the whole glorious lot of it.

2 cups (250 g) cacao butter
1 ½ cups (150 g) cacao powder
2 cups (200 g) mesquite powder
3 Tbsp agave nectar
1 tsp Etherium Pink
2 tsp suma

Melt the butter. Put all the other ingredients in another bowl, and give them a good mix together. Pour the melted butter in and give another stir. Pour the chocolate into a large tray and leave in the fridge to set for three hours. When it's done, tip out and cut into cubes, six across by five down.

Magic Manna

Makes 30 pieces
15 mins
Blender

> How much magic can you mannage?

1 ¾ cups (220 g) cacao butter
2 cups (250 g) cacao nibs
1 cup (100 g) mesquite powder
½ cup (50 g) lucuma powder
3 Tbsp agave nectar
2 Tbsp Crystal Manna or
  E3 AFA flakes

To start, melt the butter. Grind the nibs in a high-power blender*. Add the melted butter into the blender and blend again until the butter and nibs have combined. Add the mesquite, lucuma, agave nectar, and blend one more time. Once you've got a runny chocolate cream, stir in one tablespoon of the Crystal Manna. The reason for stirring it in rather than blending it in is to preserve the sparkly flakes visible in the chocolate. Pour half the chocolate into a medium-sized tray. Sprinkle the second tablespoon of Crystal Manna over the top in an even layer. Then pour the rest of the chocolate on top and leave it in the fridge to set. When it's ready, take out of the fridge and cut into cubes, five down by six across. You will have a thin line of green glitter running through the centre of your slab.

*You can use a coffee grinder to grind the nibs, but will have to transfer to a blender for the remaining steps.

Living Lavender

Makes 30 pieces
15 mins
Blender

> The quality of cacao butter available can be very variable. If it's very cheap, it's probably not food-quality, but used for cosmetic use. It's not bad for you, but it won't have much taste, and it quite likely isn't raw. Unfortunately, there is no official accreditation body yet for what is of truly raw standards, and many companies (perhaps unwittingly) try to pass goods off as raw that aren't.

1 ¼ cups (150 g) cacao butter
½ cup (75 g) coconut oil
2 cups (250 g) cacao nibs
1 cup (100 g) lucuma powder
⅓ cups (100 g) or agave nectar
1 tbsp purple corn extract
5 drops lavender oil

Melt the cacao butter and coconut oil together. Grind the nibs in a high-power blender or grinder. Put all the ingredients together in the blender and blend to a puree. Pour into a medium-sized tray and leave to set in the fridge for three hours. Once it's set, turn it out, and cut into pieces, six across by five down.

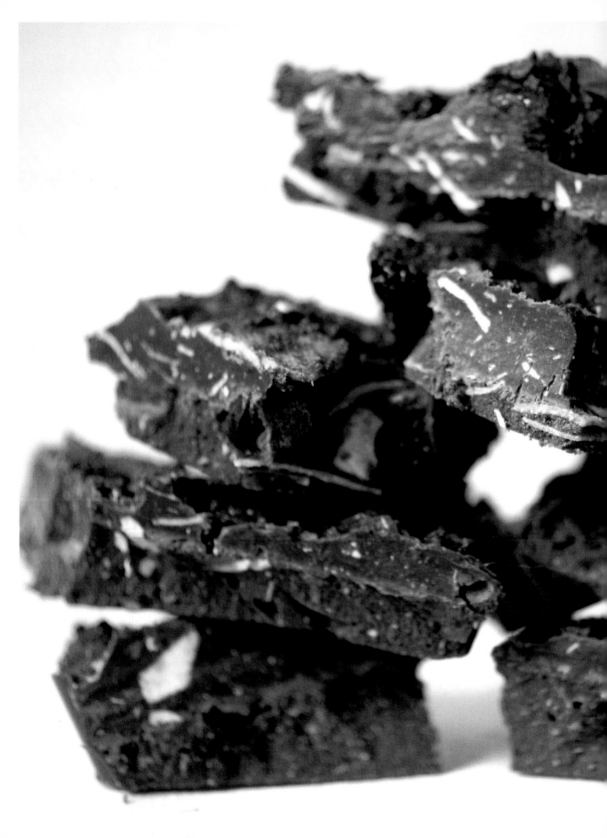

Minted

Makes 30 pieces
10 mins, 3 hours setting
No equipment needed

Peppermint is one of the most popular flavors in chocolate. We find the best method for adding flavorings is with organic essential oils. These are the purest option, and you only need a few drops to get a really quality taste. The Medicine Flower Extract Company also do an incredible range of raw flavor essences which I highly recommend checking out.

1 ½ cups (180 g) coconut oil
½ cup (60 g) cacao butter
1 ¾ cups (175 g) cacao powder
2 cups (200 g) mesquite powder
3 Tbsp agave nectar
1 Tbsp purple corn extract
2 Tbsp Crystal Manna or
    E3 AFA flakes
5 drops peppermint
1 cup (100 g) raisins
1 cup (50 g) coconut flakes

Melt the coconut oil and cacao butter together. In another bowl, put the cacao powder, mesquite, agave nectar, purple corn extract, Crystal Manna and peppermint. Give it all a good stir together, then pour in the melted butters and stir again. Add in the raisins and coconut flakes and give one final mix. Pour into a tray and leave in the fridge for three hours. When it's ready, turn it out and cut into cubes, five across by six down.

The Grass Is Always Greener

Makes 30 pieces
15 mins
No equipment needed

I love barleygrass in chocolate, it softens the stimulating effects of cacao and gives it a calmer, balanced, just plain greener edge. Yacon root is another aesthetically exciting addition to chocolate—it looks like yellow flowers in the grass, but maybe that's just me.

1 cup (125 g) coconut oil
1 cup (125 g) cacao butter
1 ½ cups (150 g) cacao powder
1 cup (100 g) mesquite powder
½ cup (50 g) barleygrass
½ cup (50 g) hemp protein powder
3 Tbsp agave nectar
1 cup (50 g) yacon root

Melt the coconut oil and cacao butter together. In a mixing bowl, stir together the cacao powder, mesquite, barleygrass and hemp protein powder so they're evenly mixed. Add the melted butters and agave nectar, and stir again. Finally stir the yacon root in thoroughly, and pour into a large tray to set. After three hours, remove it from the tray and cut into pieces, six across by five down.

Make It Mulberry

Makes 30 pieces
15 mins
Blender

Using dried mulberries to sweeten your chocolate is a great low-glycemic option that means you can avoid relying on the more processed powders and syrups to get the sweetness you desire. They also add an interesting chewy texture to your chocolate.

1 ¾ cups (230 g) cacao butter
2 cups (150 g) mulberries
1 cup (100 g) mesquite powder
1 ¾ cups (175 g) cacao powder
5 drops orange oil
1 tsp Aulterra

To start, melt the cacao butter. Mash the mulberries in a grinder or food processor until they're a paste. Put all the ingredients together in the blender, and blend to a thick cream. Pour into a large tray and leave to set in the fridge for three hours. When it's hardened, pop it out and cut it into cubes, five across by six down.

B&B

Makes 30 pieces
15 mins
No equipment needed

> Get some R&R with B&B—buckwheat and barberry—it's what my seaside town
> Brighton is all about. He Shou Wu is a tonic herb used in Chinese medicine that
> is a wonderful mood booster, as well as strengthening the inner organs.

1 cup (125 g) cacao butter
½ cup (50 g) coconut oil
1 ¾ cups (175 g) cacao powder
1 Tbsp suma
1 Tbsp he shou wu powder
½ cup (120 g) raw honey
1 cup (100 g) buckwheaties
½ cup (50 g) barberries *

Melt the cacao butter and coconut oil together first. In a mixing bowl, stir together
the cacao powder, suma, and he shou wu. Stir in the melted butters and honey and
give it another good mix. Finally stir in the buckwheaties and barberries and when
they're evenly mixed in, pour it into a large tray and leave in the fridge to set for
three hours. Once it's hard, turn it out and cut into cubes, five across by six down.

* Available at rawliving.eu/barberries-organic-dried-100g.html

Hi-Flier

Makes 20 pieces
10 mins, 2 hours setting
No equipment needed

> This chocolate is not for the faint-hearted. Intense in flavor and effects, it will take you to places you didn't know it was possible to go with chocolate. One for the hardcore faithful, you know the score.

1 ¼ cups (150 g) cacao butter
1 ¾ cups (175 g) cacao powder
⅓ cup (100 g) agave nectar
1 tsp Blue Manna or E3 AFA Mend
1 tsp Etherium Gold

Melt the butter, and once it's ready, add it to the rest of the ingredients. Give it a good stir, and pour into a small tray. Once it's set, which should only take a couple of hours, turn out and cut into pieces, four by five.

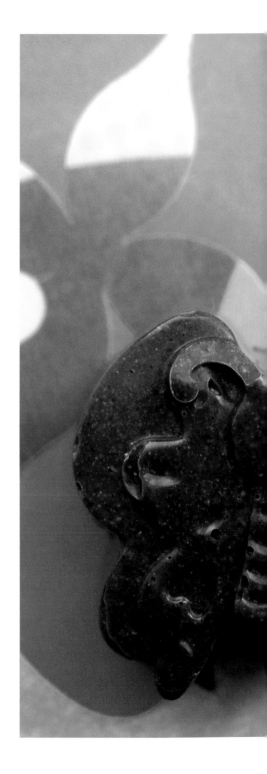

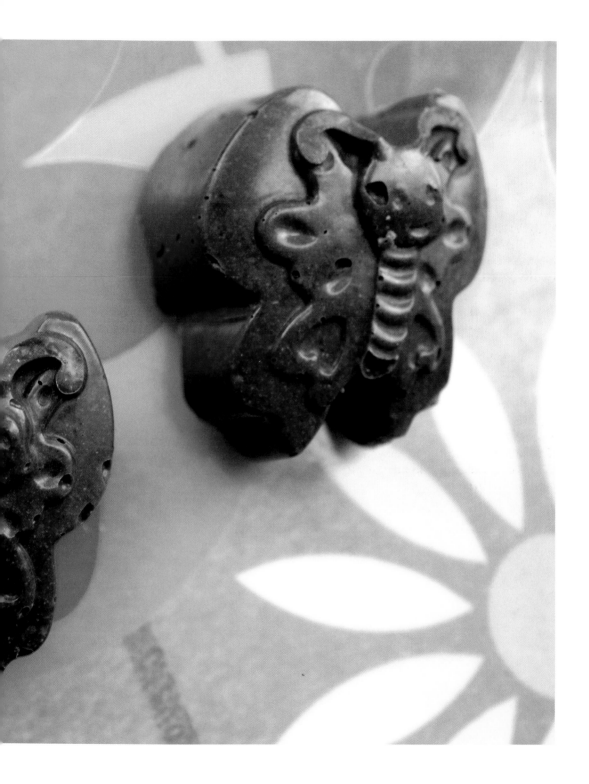

Hempster Genes

Makes 25 pieces
15 mins
Blender

This is a bit fudgier than the other chocolates because it's made with hemp seeds rather than butter. Hemp and chocolate is a very grounding combination—the protein in the hemp and the kick in the cacao make this very strengthening and energizing.

2 cups (250 g) shelled hemp seeds
2 cups (250 g) cacao nibs
4 Tbsp agave nectar

Blend the hemp seeds in a high-power blender or food grinder. Remove them from the machine, and then put the cacao nibs in and give them a good whiz. When they are completely broken down to a powder, add the hemp back in with the agave nectar, if you have a high-power blender. If not, transfer to a food processor and use that. You should end up with a sticky mass which you will need to remove with a spoon and press into a medium-sized tray. It should harden in about three hours. Cut into cubes, five by five. Will keep for up to two weeks in the fridge.

Hi-Five

Makes 30 pieces
15 mins
Blender

This was the first bar we made, along with the Hi-bar. I'm not a big eater of nuts, and the Hi-bar was made with Brazil nuts, so I wanted to do a bar that was nut-free. We called this Hi-Five because it contains five different types of seeds.

2 cups (250 g) cacao nibs
½ cup (50 g) hemp seeds
½ cup (50 g) pumpkin seeds
½ cup (50 g) sesame seeds
½ cup (50 g) sunflower seeds
⅓ cup (50 g) flaxseeds
3 Tbsp agave nectar

Grind the nibs in a high-power blender or coffee grinder. Remove from the machine, and put in all the seeds together to grind them. Then if you're using a high-power blender, either put the cacao and seeds together in that, or transfer to a food processor. Add the agave nectar and give it a good mix until you have a sticky ball. Press into a tray and leave in the fridge to set. Once it's done, cut into pieces, six down by five across. Will keep for up to two weeks in the fridge.

Hi-Seas

Makes 16 pieces
10 mins, 2 hours setting
Blender

> Seaweed and chocolate seems an unlikely combination, and people either love this or hate this. I'm a big seaweed fan and I love this because I get to eat two of my favorite foods at once.

2 cups (250 g) cacao nibs
1 cup (25 g) dulse
½ cup (60 ml) hemp oil
1 cup (120 ml) agave nectar
1 Tbsp kelp powder

Grind the nibs in a high-power blender*. Add the dulse and blend again, until the dulse is completely powdered. Add in the kelp, agave nectar and hemp oil and blend again until creamy. It's really good like this, warm and liquid straight from the blender. Press into a medium-sized tray, and leave in the fridge to set for at least two hours. Once it's ready, turn out and cut into cubes, four across by four down.

*You can use a coffee grinder to grind the nibs, but will have to transfer to a blender for the remaining steps.

Blissful Blue

Makes 30 pieces
10 mins, 3 hours setting
Blender

> In the original edition of *Raw Magic*, the intro to this recipe was about love and pain and surrender. Here, I dedicate it to my girl, the strings girl, Ysanne Spevack, who writes exquisite love songs on that very same topic, as well as being one of the most delightful ambassadors of raw chocolate you will find in the entire state of California.

1 ¾ cups (220 g) coconut oil
1 ¼ cups (150 g) cacao nibs
¾ cup (75 g) cacao powder
1 ½ cups (150 g) mesquite powder
⅓ cup (50 g) xylitol
2 tsp Blue Manna or E3 AFA Mend
2 Tbsp vanilla powder
    or 2 vanilla pods

Melt the coconut oil first. Grind up the cacao nibs until they are completely powdered—if you're using whole vanilla pods it's best to grind them up with the nibs. Add the melted butter, cacao powder, mesquite, and xylitol in now, with the vanilla if it's not already in there, and give it another good blend. Measure in the Blue Manna and blend one last time. Pour into a large tray and leave in the fridge to set for three hours. Turn out and cut into cubes, five across by six down.

Chocolate Halva

Makes 20 pieces
15 mins, 3 hours setting
Blender

Back in the day, we used to buy big 2.5 kg blocks of halva and cane them. There's something tremendously reassuring about the combination of sesame seeds and honey—add some chocolate into the mix to find divine solace in this candy.

2 cups (200 g) sesame seeds
½ cup (100 g) honey
¾ cup (75 g) cacao powder
1 Tbsp vanilla powder or extract or 1 pod
½ cup (50 g) raisins

Grind the sesame seeds in a high-power blender or grinder, keep going until they're as mashed as you can get them. If you haven't got a high-power blender, transfer them to a food processor, and add the other ingredients. If you're using a high-power blender, just add in the honey, cacao powder and vanilla. Give it a really good pounding, until all the ingredients are as amalgamated as possible, with as few traces of sesame seeds left as you can, just a ball of sticky candy. Add the raisins in and give it a half-hearted go, so that they're still discernible in the mix. Spoon out into a medium-sized tray and press down. Keep in the fridge for three hours, then turn out and cut into pieces, four across by five down. Keep stored in the fridge for up to two weeks.

Drinks

Basically, I'm spoiling you here.

Recipes are pretty superfluous when it comes to superfood drinks. Once you get into them, you'll realise that drinking them is by far the fastest, easiest and most effective way to get them into your system. Either in teas, milks, or smoothies, superfood drinks will become an unmissable part of your daily intake. And here the possibilities really are limitless. Just be guided by your intuition and use a little of everything you fancy.

Gojis? Check. Lucuma? Check. Purple corn extract? Check. We never use teabags anymore, we just freestyle it with a teaspoon of this and a pinch of that. No time for lunch? Throw your favorites in the blender with a generous serving of water, pour into a flask and take with you to drink on the go, it'll see you through easy until you have time to sit down for a big green salad.

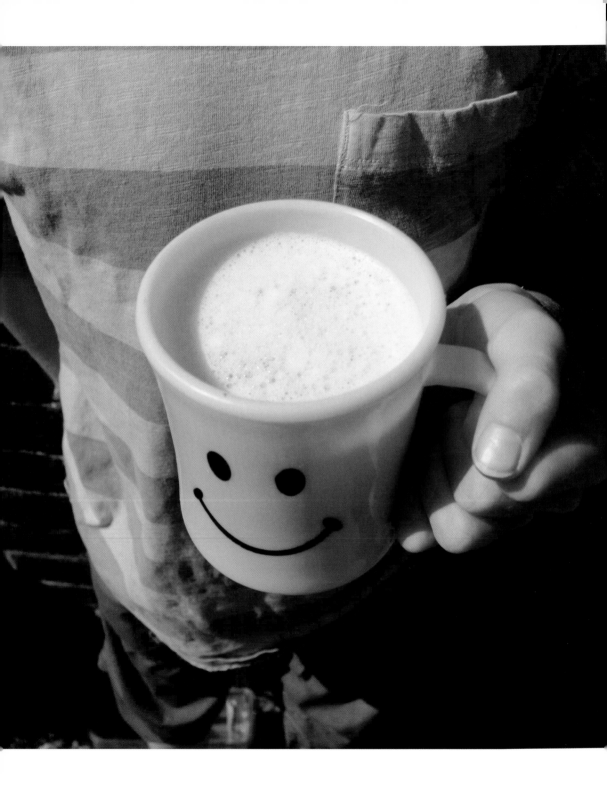

Milkalicious

Serves one
5 mins
Blender

Homemade milk doesn't come any easier. Just pop it in the blender and whiz for a minute. This works with most nuts and seeds, but hemp is our favorite for flavor and nutritional potency.

2 Tbsp shelled hemp seeds
1 cup (250 ml) water

Blend. Um, that's it, really. Just blend.

Macamilk

Serves two
Blender
5 mins

Thicker than water but thinner than smoothies, my milks are really magic. By putting superfoods into water, we help make them more absorbable, and their effects are stronger.

2 Tbsp shelled sesame seeds
2 Tbsp lucuma powder
1 Tbsp maca
1 tsp raw honey or agave nectar
2 cups (500 ml) water

Put everything in the blender and blend for two minutes or until smooth.

Beat Me Up

Serves one
5 mins
Blender

> Black and blue, this milk will slap you 'round the face a bit when you need waking up. In a very loving way, of course.

1 Tbsp cacao nibs
1 Tbsp maca powder
1 Tbsp lucuma powder
1 tsp xylitol
⅛ tsp Etherium Black
¼ tsp Blue Manna or
    E3 AFA Mend
1 cup (250 ml) water

Put everything in the blender, adding the water gradually while the blender is turning. Blend for a minute until the cacao nibs are ground down.

Heaven's Juice

Serves two
Blender
5 mins

> How could you not lead a heavenly life when you can drink this every day?

2 Tbsp shelled hemp seeds
2 Tbsp mesquite powder
1 Tbsp cacao powder
2 tsp agave nectar
2 cups (500 ml) water

Put all the ingredients in the blender and blend for a couple of minutes, or until smooth.

Purple Passion Milk

Serves one
Blender
5 mins

Who do you love? Write down the five people you know who inspire the most passion in you, and promise to share a glass of this juice with them all in the next week. Then write down five heroes and sheroes who you would love to have a purple passion party with and dream of it in the boring spaces when you're washing up or waiting in line at the grocery store.

2 Tbsp shelled hemp seeds
1 tsp purple corn extract
¼ tsp suma
1 Tbsp raw honey or agave nectar
1 cup (250 ml) water

Put all your ingredients in the blender and blend for two minutes, or until smooth.

Barley Blaster

Serves two
5 mins
Blender

This will turn you into a lean, green peace-making machine.

2 Tbsp barleygrass powder
2 Tbsp shelled hemp seeds
1 tsp cacao powder
¼ tsp purple corn extract
1 lemon, juiced
pinch salt
2 cups (500 ml) water

Put everything in the blender, with half of the water. Blend the lot up and gradually add the rest of the water. The result should be thinner than a smoothie, thicker than milk. Drink immediately.

Spiral Tribe

Serves two
10 mins
Blender

Who'd have thought to name a smoothie after an early 1990s sound system that she used to squat with in South London? Oh, that'll be me. Spiral Tribe in the area, make some fucking noise…

1 pear
1 banana
1 Tbsp spirulina
2 dates
1 cup (250 ml) water

Quarter the pear, removing the stem and the pips. Peel the banana and break it into quarters. Put all the ingredients apart from the water in the blender and blend for a minute so the fruits are broken down. Then gradually add the water while the blender is turning.

Camu Get Me

Serves two
5 mins
Blender

A bit like goji pudding (p. 167) without the pudding.

1 Tbsp camu camu
½ cup (50 g) goji berries
2 Tbsp lucuma powder
1 Tbsp agave nectar
1 lemon, juiced
½ cup (25 g) coconut flakes
3 cups (750 ml) water

Put everything apart from the water in the blender and give it a good whiz. Keep it turning and add the water gradually. Once it's all in, give it another 10 seconds and it'll be ready.

Perhaps He's Perfect

Serves two
5 mins, presoaking 4 hours
Blender

Yeah, you know, I really think he is. There's nothing about him I would change—the ups and the downs, when he's pushing me away, when he's pulling me close, when he's here, when he's gone, when we're alone, when we're at a party, when we're hanging out, when we're really hectic, when we're talking, when we're sitting in silence, when we're working, when we're playing, I love it all, all of the time.

2 Tbsp almonds, soaked 4–8 hours
2 Tbsp bee pollen
2 Tbsp gojis
2 tsp agave nectar
2 cups (500 ml) water

Presoak the almonds for at least one hour, preferably overnight. Put everything in the blender and add the water gradually, as the blender is running. Blend for two minutes, until there are no bits of almond left.

Goji Orgasm

Serves one
5 mins
Blender

If you want to get cosmic, you have to stop worrying about the "hows" of life. Knowing what you want, focusing on the goals, and just trusting in the universe to deliver, leaving the details to the divine intelligence to negotiate, creates space for the outrageous to happen and the universe to blow your mind. This smoothie will put you into that space where you don't care how, you just know, and that's the way it is.

⅔ cup (60 g) gojis
⅓ cup (30 g) almonds
⅓ cup (30 g) cacao nibs
1 ½ cups (400 ml) water

Put the gojis, almonds and nibs in the blender, and add the water gradually, really slow or it will end up bitty. Keep whizzing for a couple of minutes until it's smooth. Drink, and then make sure you've got lots to do—you'll be buzzing for hours.

My Chocolate Kingdom

Serves one
5 mins
Blender

It's an Edward Monkton card—"they brought me great **MOUNTAINS** of **CHOCOLATE** and thereof I did eat. And it did not make me feel **ILL** or **ASHAMED**, neither did it put weight on my **THIGHS**. For the chocolate was health-giving and **NOURISH-ING**, and the more I ate, the more **BEAUTIFUL** I became." This man knows. Edmund, if you're reading this, let us have your address, and we'll send you some chocolate, maybe not a mountain but a generous amount, you know.

½ cup (60 g) macadamias
2 Tbsp cacao powder
1 Tbsp mesquite powder
1 Tbsp lucuma powder
1 Tbsp xylitol
1 ½ cups (400 ml) water

Put everything but the water in the blender. Start off with half the water; adding the rest in gradually, as the blender is running. Blend for a few minutes until there are no lumps of nut left.

Macoffee

Serves one
2 mins
Kettle

Maca's malty taste lends itself well to hot drinks. This gives you a boost, just like coffee but with none of the side effects. If you are worried about overheating your maca with boiling water, you have a few alternatives. You can flick the kettle off a minute before it boils, heat your water in a pan to the right temperature, or do as I did and invest in a kettle with temperature control so you can heat your water without boiling it. Ideally you want water heated to 176° F.

1 tsp maca powder
pinch crystal salt
1 tsp agave nectar
1 ⅓ cups (330 ml) water

Put the maca, salt and agave nectar in a cup and add hot water.

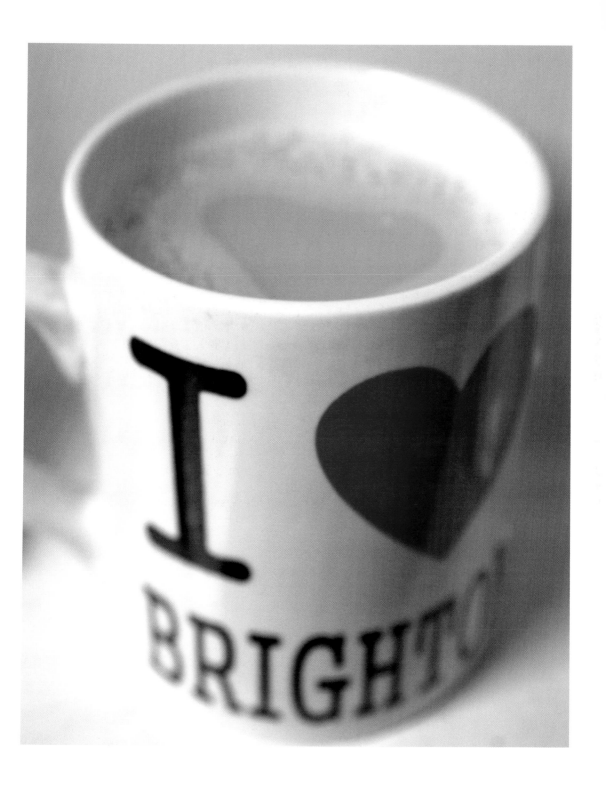

Witch's Tea

Serves one
2 mins
Kettle

> This purple and green brew is sure to cast a spell on everyone who drinks it.

½ tsp purple corn extract
¼ tsp blue-green algae
1 tsp agave nectar
pinch salt
2 cups (500 ml) water

Put the purple corn extract, algae, agave nectar and salt into a cup. Pour over water heated to around 176° F (see p. 250). This tea is quite strong, so you can make top-ups with it: when you've drunk half the cup, top up with more water, and do this every time until it's too diluted to drink anymore. You can usually get at least three top-ups from a cup.

Wizard's Tea

Serves one
5 mins
Kettle

> This tea is warming, revitalizing, cleansing, and third-eye activating! What more could you want from a cuppa?

¼ tsp purple corn extract
¼ tsp dried chili flakes
juice ¼ lemon
1 cup (250 ml) water

Heat the water (see p. 250). Put purple corn extract, chili and lemon in cup and add hot water.

Mayan Tea

Serves one
2 mins
Kettle

Chocolate was originally consumed by the Aztecs as a hot drink, mixed with vanilla and chili.

½ tsp cacao powder
½ tsp dried chili flakes
pinch salt
2 cups (500 ml) water

Put the cacao powder, flakes and salt in a cup. Fill with heated water (p. 250). This is a strong drink—you can get a few top-ups out of it. When you've drunk half a cup, refill with hot water, and it will still taste good. You can usually do this three or four times before it starts getting too diluted.

Superbeing Tea

Serves one
5 mins
Kettle

When you feel the world is a harsh and lonely place, make yourself a cup of this and feel re-inspired to enter the battle and fight for your right to live in the light.

1 tsp maca powder
½ tsp cacao powder
1 tsp lucuma powder
pinch salt
2 cups (500 ml) water

Boil the kettle. Put everything in a cup and pour half the water in. When you've drunk half the tea, top it up with some more water—you can do this two or three times and it still tastes great.

Go Tea

Serves one
5 mins
Kettle

No, not a jazz-head beard, a tea to make you smile. Gojis in your tea is the best thing since...the gojis you had in your breakfast cereal, probably.

1 Tbsp goji berries
½ tsp cacao powder
1 tsp mesquite powder
pinch salt
1 cup (250 ml) water

Heat the water (p. 250). Put all the ingredients in the cup and pour the water in. Some of the gojis slurp into your mouth when you first start drinking and some get left at the bottom and get all plump and moist....

Budgeting

People often worry that the raw food diet is going to be expensive, and it certainly can be: there is no shortage of little bottles available costing $50 a pop. However, the way we do the raw food diet can be very economical. I recommend that your diet is based around 50% local seasonal organic vegetables, by volume. Buying local and seasonal is always more economical than buying imported produce. If you include a lot of sprouts and indoor greens, you're ensuring your food is local, seasonal, and organic! And it costs pennies to sprout and grow greens. I don't eat a lot of nuts as I find them congesting, and hard to digest. Seeds, on the other hand, are better for the body and a lot more economical—seeds are often as little as a quarter of the price of nuts.

As far as the superfoods go, it may seem that some of them carry a hefty price tag. But remember two things: first, I recommend that you take superfoods in very small doses. If you're purchasing reishi extract, for instance, I would recommend just consuming ¼ teaspoon in a day to begin with. That means, if you're buying a 100 g jar of reishi extract, it will last you at least 50 days. As it's unlikely that you will actually remember to include it every day, you are looking at around two to three months to use up the jar. When you divide it up into daily doses like that, suddenly it doesn't seem so costly. I do recommend with superfoods that, at first at least, you just work with a few at a time—choose three to five that you most resonate with and work with those until you get to understand how they work with your body and mind. There is no point going out and buying everything at once, because your body won't know what has hit it!

Second, the vitality that taking these products gives us cannot be measured in money. People spend fortunes on alcohol, tobacco, and home entertainment systems to help them pass the days. The buzz we get from eating superfoods is greater than any recreational substance such as beer or cigarettes, and far more economical when you compare them directly. And whereas those substances deplete your energy, and make you feel worse after the effects have worn off, the superfoods increase your energy a hundredfold. Who can put a price on that magical idea you had after your raw chocolate breakfast smoothie, or the extra two hours of quality time you gained from having a superfood-filled dinner? At one of my talks once, a man said to me that he didn't mind spending a bit extra on superfoods because it made him feel so abundant. And because he felt abundant, he was attracting more good stuff into his life and so it was worth the extra investment.

As far as superfoods go, as I've mentioned, I don't believe it's necessary to go all out and get everything all at once. Better to start off with a few and work up gradually. I would recommend focusing on the green powders (spirulina, chlorella, Klamath Lake algae, barleygrass, wheatgrass and hemp protein) and adaptogens (aloe vera, maca, suma, reishi, ashwagandha), and just taking one or two from each group to begin.

The main superfoods I use on a daily basis, aside from the green powders and adaptogens, are shelled hemp, goji berries, and chia. I also love MSM, which is a naturally occurring form of the mineral sulphur.

Substitution

Raw food cuisine is much freer than more traditional methods of food preparation. There are many fewer ways you can mess it up, and many more opportunities for creativity. You can't burn anything, for a start!

Never be worried about tampering with a recipe to suit your immediate needs. It's often the way to discover a new favorite combination. Here are some examples of ingredients that can be interchanged. Obviously, the finished recipe won't be the same. But it won't be a failure, just different—and maybe better, who knows?

Shopping List

Please note that some of the ingredients in the recipes you may find hard to track down. So often, people pick up a bag of lucuma or maca because they've heard it's good for them, and then don't know what to do with it! So I wanted to share these recipes with you to encourage you to use these new and often unfamiliar foods and experience their benefits in your life. But maybe you've picked up this book, and now you're struggling to find out where you can buy sea spaghetti or mulberries. I believe that they are all such wonderful foods, that as more people discover them and they become more popular, they will become more commonplace. Raw food shops, cafés, restaurants and online stores are sprouting up (pun intended!) all over the world right now. Your local health food store should be your first port of call. If you can't find what you're looking for there, it's always worth requesting if they can get it in. Small independent stores generally love to be able to please their customers and cater to their needs. And the more they hear that people are requesting a particular item, the more likely they are to start carrying it in store. If they can't help you, our company Raw Living (rawliving.eu) stocks everything you need. We are based in Europe, but you may be surprised how low the shipping charges are to the USA. In Europe, we are always importing new raw food and superfood products from the USA. Why don't you reverse the trend, and import some from Europe! If you are based in America, and want to use an American store, there are many raw online stores to choose from. I recommend Raw Guru (rawguru.com), which also has a ton of helpful info, recipes and interviews.

I believe a good raw food diet is around 50% organic local seasonal vegetables, by volume. The most nutritious vegetables, and often the most economical to purchase, are the green leafy vegetables.

The rest of the diet should be comprised of:

Fruits: again, local, seasonal and organic wherever possible. Dried fruits should be used minimally because they can unbalance the blood sugar and damage the teeth.

Sprouts: we sprout wheat, buckwheat, oats, quinoa, mung beans, chickpeas, adzuki beans, lentils, sunflower seeds, alfalfa seeds, radish seeds and broccoli seeds.

Indoor Greens: so easy to do—even easier than sprouting I think, and the best way to make sure your food is local and seasonal. You can grow hemp (outside of the USA), flax, chia, yellow pea shoots, gojis, sunflower seeds and buckwheat greens very easily.

Fermented Foods: such as sauerkraut, kimchi, raw cheeses and yogurts (either seed-based or dairy-based), kefir and kombucha.

Sea Vegetables: dulse, nori, sea spaghetti, kelp, kelp noodles, arame, hijiki, wakame.

Herbs and Spices: are essential for turning a plain dish into something special. *Fresh*: ginger, garlic, red chili peppers, parsley, cilantro, dill, basil, rosemary. *Dried*: cinnamon, cumin, coriander, paprika, cayenne, turmeric, oregano, thyme, vanilla.

Nuts: walnuts, almonds, cashews, coconut (fresh or dried), Brazils, hazelnuts, pecans, pine nuts, macadamias.

Seeds: sesame, sunflower, pumpkin, hemp, flax, chia.

Oils: flax, chia and hemp oils are raw, but other cold-pressed oils aren't, necessarily. When buying olive oil, make sure it's extra virgin. It's handy to get some raw nut and seed butters in as well.

Sweeteners: Agave, yacon syrup, unpasteurized honey, lucuma, mesquite, carob, xylitol, coconut palm sugar, stevia. I don't think there is a perfect raw sweetener. Much agave, coconut palm sugar, and yacon syrup available isn't even raw. Best to use them all in small amounts, and not rely on any one too heavily. Yacon and stevia are the only two that are suitable for candida sufferers and diabetics.

Miso: get unpasteurized. Although not strictly a raw food, because of the enzymatic activity, it is a living food, and very beneficial for the immune system.

Tamari or shoyu: these are also Japanese fermented foods. Tamari has a more intense flavor, shoyu is slightly mellower. Whenever I have specified tamari in a recipe, shoyu can be substituted if you prefer. I use tamari because it is wheat-free.

Braggs Liquid Aminos: this is a raw product, but is best used in moderation, as it contains naturally occurring monosodium glutamate.

Salt: any crystal rock salt is good. Himalayan salt is very popular. I like to pick up local sea salts wherever I travel.

Vinegars: unpasteurized apple cider vinegar is raw. There is also a raw coconut vinegar. I do love a good balsamic vinegar or rice vinegar, although these are not raw.

Glossary

Sprouted/Dried Buckwheat
Buckwheat is technically a seed, not a grain, and it doesn't contain gluten. It is very alkalizing. If you see buckwheaties in a recipe, that means buckwheat that has been soaked, sprouted and dehydrated.

Purple Corn Extract
Make sure to buy the extract, not the flour. Purple corn extract is high in antioxidants, gently stimulates the pineal gland, and turns your food and drinks purple!

Crystal Manna or E3 AFA Flakes
This is a potentiated form of Klamath Lake blue-green algae. Klamath Lake algae is a complete food, containing all the nutrients the body needs.

Blue Manna
Blue Manna is an extract of blue-green algae, which is pure PEA. PEA is good for focus, concentration, and improving mood.

Mulberries
You can get white mulberries or black mulberries. They are a low-glycemic sweet treat.

Suma
Suma is a South American adaptogenic root, used to rebalance the body. Use sparingly, it's very potent!

Mucuna
Mucuna is one of my personal favorites. It's high in L-Dopa, the precursor to dopamine, and 5-htp, the precursor to serotonin. Both of these are natural mood-boosting chemicals.

Cacao Butter
The oil from the cacao bean. An essential ingredient in raw chocolate making.

He Shou Wu
A Chinese tonifying herb, strengthening, nurturing and mood-boosting. Also reputedly good for hair growth!

Irish Moss
A gelatinous seaweed used to set mousses, desserts, cakes and pies. Careful preparation is needed, but once you get the hang of it, the results are wonderful.

Ashwagandha
An Ayurvedic adaptogenic herb, which is subtly strengthening and centering. Particularly good for men.

Aulterra
A monatomic trace extract from the seabed, which has been proven to activate DNA.

Yacon Root
Yacon is suitable for people suffering from candida or diabetes as the sugars in it are not recognized by the body. Yacon root is a dried snack, similar in taste to dried apple or pineapple.

Mushroom Powders

Medicinal mushrooms are one of the very best things for your immune system because of the polysaccharides they contain. Some examples are reishi, cordyceps, chaga, lion's mane.

Etherium Gold, Black, Pink, Red Monatomic Trace Elements

Please see page 65 for more info.

Hemp Butter

Like peanut butter, this is a hemp seed paste. Best source of vegetarian protein.

Klamath Lake Blue-Green Algae

Grows wild in Oregon. Please see page 49 for more info.

Coconut Oil

The fat from the coconut. Antibacterial, antimicrobial, balances the metabolism, easy to digest, best dietary source of lauric acid.

Flaxseeds

High in the essential fatty acid omega-3. Balances the gut. Makes the best raw crackers!

Hemp (shelled only)

Whole hemp seeds are available in Europe, but not in the USA and Canada. The shelled seeds are white and nutty in flavor and have many uses in raw cuisine. Hemp is one of the most amazing plants on the planet, with a multitude of uses.

Chia

Best dietary source of omega-3s. Will absorb up to four times their volume in liquids, making them economical to use. Very energizing.

Raw Cacao Powder

This is the cacao solids, with the fats removed. Incredible source of antioxidants.

Raw Cacao Nibs

These are simply the beans which have been shelled and broken into small pieces.

Lucuma Powder

Lucuma is a Peruvian fruit, used as a low-glycemic sweetener, which has a biscuit-like flavor.

Mesquite Powder

Mesquite is a low-glycemic sweetener from the same family as carob. It has a caramelly flavor.

Bee Pollen

Produced by the flowers, harvested by the bees, pollen is a perfect food, containing every nutrient the body needs.

Camu Camu

An Amazonian berry which is very rich in vitamin C and has a lemony flavor.

Maca

A Peruvian root vegetable which is good for energy and stamina.

Coconut Palm Sugar

A low-glycemic sweetener with a beautiful flavor. Most coconut sugars on the market aren't raw.

Raw Honey
Try and get local honey if possible. Good raw honey produced by an individual beekeeper is a world apart from mass-produced commercial honeys.

Agave Nectar
A syrup from the same cactus plant that tequila comes from. Be sure to purchase high quality agave to be sure it's raw.

Xylitol
Low-glycemic sweetener made from fermented birch bark. Not all xylitol is raw, check with your supplier.

Coconut Flakes
Dried coconut pieces.

Hemp Protein
The protein extract from the seeds. Best vegetarian source of protein.

Spirulina
Blue-green algae, excellent source of minerals and protein.

Barleygrass
Barleygrass is similar to wheatgrass but has a much more pleasant flavor. It is extremely alkalizing.

Dulse
One of the easiest sea vegetables to get along with. Needs no soaking, just a little rinsing first.

Kelp Powder
Kelp is the most mineral-rich sea vegetable. Use in small amounts.

Vanilla Powder
The easiest way to use vanilla, vanilla powder is simply ground-down pods. Vanilla and chocolate are best friends!

Goji Berries
Antioxidant-, vitamin- and mineral-rich Chinese longevity berry. Especially good in tea.

Books

Eat Smart, Eat Raw by Kate Wood
Raw Living by Kate Wood
Ecstatic Beings by Kate Magic & Shazzie
Naked Chocolate by Shazzie & David Wolfe
Maca by Beth Ley
Wild Blue-Green Algae by Gillian McKeith
Primordial Food by Christian Drapeau
The Healing Powers of Pollen by Patrice Percie du Sert
Seven Health Secrets from the Hive by Charles H. Robson
The Wheatgrass Book by Anne Wigmore
Fats That Heal, Fats That Kill by Udo Erasmus
Superfoods by David Wolfe
Adaptogens by David Winston & Steven Maimes
The Hidden Messages from Water by Masaru Emoto
Living Magically by Gill Edwards
Excuse Me, Your Life is Waiting by Lynne Grabhorn
The Power of Now by Eckhart Tolle
Be Here Now by Ram Dass
The Field by Lynne McTaggart
Spontaneous Evolution by Bruce H. Lipton & Steve Bhaerman
Molecules of Emotion by Candace Pert
Anastasia Chronicles by Vladimir Megré
Love Without End: Jesus Speaks by Glenda Green

Kate Magic tours extensively teaching classes and workshops on raw food. Check her websites rawliving.eu and katesmagicbubble.com for information on upcoming dates.

Rawliving.eu is Europe's largest raw foods and superfoods online store. You can find everything you need there for the raw food lifestyle, as well as recipes and helpful information.

Katesmagicbubble.com is Kate's subscription website. Join for exclusive recipes, articles, videos, interviews, and the opportunity to ask Kate your questions and have them answered on the site. Plus all subscribers qualify for shopping discounts at Raw Living.

Index